To my beloved Grandma Rose, and to all the other Grandma Roses out there, I pray that the principles contained in The Great Physician's Rx for Cancer *will make a profound difference in your life.*

CONTENTS

INTRODUCTION

My Rose

I lost Grandma Rose to cancer not long ago.

She was my last surviving grandparent, and as I helplessly watched cancer emaciate this once vibrant woman to a skeleton-like seventy pounds, I sat by her bedside and recited poetry, read Scripture, and sang worship songs. I felt helpless as her bladder cancer—like a slow-moving army—invaded her body, plundered her mind, and would eventually snuff out the burning embers of nearly eighty-three years of life.

While monitoring her labored breathing, I became very emotional as I recalled the memories that bonded us closely together. At the age of twenty, when I faced my own life-and-death struggle with horrible abdominal and digestive tract diseases, I stayed with Grandma Rose from time to time when my parents needed a break from caring for me. My nurturing grandmother gently pressed a cool cloth to my feverish forehead, spooned homemade chicken soup into my mouth, and cleaned up soiled bedsheets without complaint. When I was hospitalized twice, she insisted on sleeping in a spare bed next to me. Although it wasn't funny at the time, we shared a laugh one night after a nurse slipped into my room at 4:00 a.m. and wrapped a tourniquet around Grandma Rose's left arm, thinking she was drawing blood from the patient.

Grandma Rose would have done anything for me—even give a pint of blood. What a remarkable woman! Born in 1922 in a pastoral Polish village that could have doubled as the set for *Fiddler on the Roof,* Rose was the youngest of seven children born to Gidalia and Simma Catz. An extra hand was always appreciated around the family farm. Her father owned a mill where they pressed poppy seeds and flaxseeds into oil. A tasty treat in those days was gathering the pressed seeds and patting them into hard cakes, which were dipped into *schmaltz,* the rendered fat from chicken soup.

Her Jewish family faced growing harassment during that uneasy era following World War I. Her oldest brother, Sydney, was persecuted horribly in the Polish Army. Great-grandma Simma helped Sydney escape from the Polish military, and her family arranged for his safe passage to the United States. Waiting for him at Ellis Island were several uncles and aunts who had immigrated to America.

War clouds thickened over Europe in the 1930s. When Adolf Hitler was elected chancellor of Germany in 1933, he moved quickly to pass repressive anti-Jewish laws—and brutally enforce them with his Brownshirts. Amid this hostile environment, Jewish persecution intensified elsewhere throughout Europe. Fortunately thirteen-year-old Rose joined her parents and several siblings and immigrated in 1935 to the United States, where the family settled in Queens, New York. They were among the last wave of European Jews to arrive in America prior to World War II.

Two older sisters, Sonya and Dora, who were married with their own families, stayed behind in Poland, which was not a good place to be if you happened to be Jewish in 1939. Following the

Nazi *blitzkrieg,* her sisters and their families were rounded up and shipped off to the death camps. No *Schindler's List* could save them. We believe that Rose's sisters and families were murdered inside the gas chambers of Auschwitz.

After the war, Rose married Alvin Menlowe, an immigrant from Czechoslovakia. She gave birth to my mother, Phyllis, and a younger daughter, Debbie. When I came along twenty-five years later, I was a colicky child who cut into my parents' sleeping time. Grandma Rose, who stayed with us periodically, would hide behind my crib when the lights were turned out. Then she would reach out her hand and stroke my forehead. "Jordi, Jordi . . . it's okay," she soothed. "I'm here."

Another early memory of her happened when I was two years old. Grandma Rose took me to Miami Beach—the first time I saw the ocean. My grandmother hugged me to her chest and ran us into the light surf, which scared me half to death. I'm told that I cried, but that quickly changed as I got used to the churning ocean. I soon loved wading into the warm Atlantic waters, holding the hand of the grandmother I loved.

HOOKED ON SWEETS

My parents were vegetarians until I was four years old, when my mom became pregnant with my sister, Jenna. The honor of handing me my first chicken leg went to Grandma Rose.

My grandmother didn't eat as healthy as my parents, though. At lunchtime, for instance, she happily consumed glazed doughnuts and coffee ice cream, chased with a cup of sugared coffee.

She had become hooked on sweets not long after her ship docked at Ellis Island: America, for my grandmother and her family, was the land of the free and the home of the white bread. She had heard that our streets were paved with chocolate, and cheery vendors handed out double-scoop cones on every street corner. Although she managed to eat somewhat healthier in her later years, she never lost her sweet tooth.

Her husband and my grandfather, Al, was partial to junk food as well. Perhaps that's why he suddenly died of a heart attack at the age of fifty-five when I was just eighteen months old. Grandma Rose lived as a widow and never remarried.

In early 1999, she began experiencing unusual health problems—fainting spells, excruciating stomach pains, and rampant nausea. Grandma Rose was never one to run to the doctor— that was the Old Country mind-set working—but even she knew something was terribly wrong. Doctors conducted a series of tests, including CAT scans, but they all returned negative. Her doctors were at a loss to deliver a diagnosis.

Meanwhile, Grandma Rose visited her other daughter, Debbie, who had married a chiropractor, Dr. Jim DiBlasi. They lived in Atlanta. On this occasion, she felt so weak that she had to be lifted out of bed and assisted in and out of the bathroom. The searing abdominal pains and long periods of nausea became unbearable. In her desperation, she asked her son-in-law to fetch her some pills so that she could "end it all."

Under such dire circumstances, she agreed to allow surgeons to perform emergency exploratory surgery. Doctors sliced open her abdomen and uncovered several malignant tumors tucked underneath her internal organs, which explained why her cancer had not been detected before. Doctors excised two cancerous ovaries, portions of her large and small intestines, and a malignant mass near her appendix.

Afterward, her doctors delivered the bad news to the family: Grandma Rose may not have long to live. They couldn't give us a time frame, however. My father immediately searched for the best alternative cancer clinics around the world, but each had something in common: they were all superexpensive. Grandma Rose didn't have a nest egg to cash in; she had been living off a six-hundred-dollar Social Security check each month, which was augmented by financial help from my parents and other family members. Bottom line: she couldn't afford anything that wasn't covered by Medicare.

At this time Grandma Rose asked me for help. After I recovered from my rash of debilitating diseases, I studied naturopathic medicine, nutrition, and natural therapies. When Grandma Rose was struck by cancer, I formulated a plan to regain her health—a plan that's contained in the seven keys that comprise this book, *The Great Physician's Rx for Cancer.*

Instead of slowly sinking toward death, Grandma Rose experienced a complete—and dramatic—recovery as she switched from a sugar-laden, high-carbohydrate diet to one filled with organic fruits, vegetables, and meats, supplemented with living nutrients and superfoods. Her doctors expressed amazement when follow-up CAT scans revealed she was cancer-free. She regained weight, and her energy level picked up. Her recovery allowed her to fulfill a dream of hers—and mine—when she attended my wedding. At the reception, guests clapped when Grandma Rose and I did the fox-trot to a song I had sung and recorded just for her—"Just the Way You Look Tonight," made famous by one of her favorite singers, Frank Sinatra.

For five years, Grandma Rose was the picture of health. She spoke with me at an "Overcoming Cancer" conference, joined me for television interviews following the release of my first two books, and couldn't wait for Nicki to get pregnant so that she could hold her great-grandson.

Then a couple of years ago, Grandma Rose abandoned her healthy diet as she grew complacent about her "good health." I urged her to eat better, but she didn't heed my words. When cancer revisited her, Grandma Rose *did* listen to me again. We thought we were making good progress until the day she tripped and fell down a staircase at my home, badly bruising her head and shattering her elbow on our marble floor.

She never fully recovered from that tumbling fall as her cancer returned with a vengeance. This time around, however, Grandma Rose couldn't summon the energy to fight the deadly disease. She lacked the will to continue the program I gave her.

When I learned of her grave condition, I dropped everything to be with her, flying from my residence in Palm Beach Gardens, Florida, to Aunt Debbie's home in Atlanta. There was nothing anyone could do for her.

"Grandma, would you mind if I sang to you?" I asked.

She nodded her head weakly.

I sang "I Will Be Here," a Steven Curtis Chapman song I had performed at my sister's wedding, and "Love Song" by Third Day.

I stroked her hair, told her how much she meant to me, that I loved her and would miss her more than she would ever know.

I witnessed the moment Grandma Rose was released from the bonds of this earth, and I still believe somehow that she could still be with us. That's why I've dedicated this book to her memory, praying that the principles undergirding *The Great Physician's Rx for Cancer* will make a difference in your life and/or the life of someone you love.

STILL A DEADLY DISEASE

Back in Grandma Rose's day, people spoke in hushed tones when news ran through the neighborhood that someone had been diagnosed with cancer. "The Big C," they called it, a sign of respect for the dreaded killer. People greatly feared cancer because (1) few symptoms were noticed until the deadly disease was quite advanced, and (2) doctors lacked the technology to detect the uncontrolled growth of abnormal cells in the body.

Unfortunately death-by-cancer stories like Grandma Rose's are way too common these days because "The Big C" has made a grim comeback. In 2005, the American Cancer Society announced that cancer had surpassed heart disease as the number one killer of Americans under the age of eighty-five, which comprise 98.4 percent of the population. This development has occurred during the federal government's three-decade War on Cancer, which has poured more than $50 billion into research, on top of the billions that private industry has kicked in. Despite the concerted scientific effort, about 1.4 million *new* cases of cancer were diagnosed in 2005, and approximately 570,000 died from the lethal disease. While one's eyes tend to glaze over from so many numbers, the stark reality is that half of all American men and one-third of American women will develop some type of cancer during their lifetimes.[1]

The deadliest form of cancer is lung cancer, which kills around 160,000 Americans a year—more than breast cancer, colon cancer, and prostate cancer combined. Sixty percent of patients die within a year of diagnosis. Lung cancer struck out the former smoker ABC anchorman Peter Jennings, and 87 percent of all lung cancer cases arise from those who stubbed their cigarette butts in ashtrays. Yet nonsmokers are not immune either: Dana Reeve, widow of Hollywood actor Christopher Reeve, died of lung cancer at the age of forty-four in 2005.

These grim stories of human tragedy underline the fatal qualities of cancer, which has leapfrogged past heart disease as our country's top killer. To be sure, cancer is a disease that preys on the old: about 77 percent of all cancers are diagnosed in people fifty-five years of age or older.[2] Yet cancer's icy tentacles can attack at any age. Leukemia, a type of blood cancer, is a known child killer, while breast cancer has buried too many mothers of young children. In addition, cancer is an equal opportunity disease, striking Americans of all racial and ethnic groups, although the rate of cancer occurrence can vary from group to group.

This modern-day plague is a worrisome disease—and elicits feelings of dread and concern.

Fortunately, advancements in modern medicine can protect us from the ravages of cancer, and breathtaking changes in surgical techniques and radiation and chemotherapy treatments have vastly improved the chances of survivability. The five-year survival rate for most cancers is 85 percent, a result tagged to regular cancer screening.

Although improving survival rates are comforting, cancer remains a ruthless killer. For those who survive and experience remission (and lose all their hair as well as their sense of taste), the slash-and-burn cure can be worse than the disease. Modern cancer treatment revolves around two extremely unpleasant options: radiation and chemotherapy. That's why I feel deeply for anyone who could *remotely* have this disease. I have difficultly imagining the private horror of what it must be like sitting across the desk from an oncologist, nervously working a Kleenex in your hands, anxiously waiting for the verdict. What do people think after the doctor glances at the medical reports, stiffly clears his throat, and wearily announces, "I regret to inform you that you have cancer"?

I hope to spare you—and myself—from ever hearing those life-changing words, and I believe *The Great Physician's Rx for Cancer* offers you a straight path to minimize the considerable risk that you may one day develop cancer in your body. If you *have* heard those same words directed to you, then please know that you have my complete sympathy. The phrase "I know what you're going through" is not applicable here because I *don't* know what it's like to be told that I have cancer. This is one disease where an ounce of prevention is worth far more than a ton of cure, to quote an old proverb.

It's my prayer that the principles I shared with Grandma

Rose, combined with sound medical advice, will send your cancer on a remission trip and never return.

A RAY OF HOPE

Although gloomy news and cancer travel in pairs, I have encouraging news to report. The incidence of death from cancer has fallen steadily in the United States since the 1990s, according to a major American Cancer Society study.[3] Death rates from all cancers combined—lung, colon, breast, and prostate—dropped 1.1 percent each year from 1993 to 2001, falling around 10 percent during that time. Leading cancer specialists say that aggressive prevention, earlier detection, and improved treatment have improved survival rates.

The focus of *The Great Physician's Rx for Cancer* will be on aggressive prevention since the best way to survive cancer is never to get the disease in the first place. I believe that following the seven keys contained in *The Great Physician's Rx for Cancer* could keep this awful disease, which claims more than 1,500 lives every day, at arm's length.

No matter how well you eat, how many times a week you exercise, or how many precautions you take regarding the toxins in your environment, cancer can rear its ugly head through no fault of your own (although your lifestyle accounts for nearly two-thirds of all cancers, as you'll soon learn). As Scripture says, "He makes His sun rise on the evil and on the good, and sends rain on the just and on the unjust" (Matt. 5:45).

The presence of cancer in you or a family member isn't an

indication of sin in your life, just as a car accident wouldn't point to that either. Cancer happens, and the illness is as old as Genesis. The oldest known descriptions of this deadly disease are found in writings from the ancient Egyptians, where tumors of the breast were described. Hippocrates, the Greek physician (460–370 B.C.), is believed to be the first person to distinguish between benign and malignant tumors.[4] The development of anesthesia in the mid-1800s gave doctors the ability to cut out and remove tumors, but it wasn't until a century ago that better microscopes allowed doctors to actually see how cancer cells were markedly different than the surrounding normal cells.

Every medical school student learns that cancer is a disease of the human cells caused by a breakdown in the immune system. The entire human body is comprised of cells, which, by definition, contain genetic material (or DNA) that tells the cells what to do. In a healthy body, cells divide at a controlled rate in order to grow and repair damaged tissues and replace dying cells. The body quickly recognizes any abnormal cells and removes them before they can present harm.

Cells are constantly dividing and growing; these around-the-clock activities keep us in good health. When the body cannot check the growth of abnormal cells, however, these "bad" cells keep multiplying until a mass of tissue, called a growth or tumor, slowly emerges. Think of the entire process as something akin to stepping on an ant pile and watching an army of angry ants attack any skin in sight.

Tumors are either benign or malignant. While benign tumors

are often no more than nuisances, the term *malignant* strikes fear in our hearts because that means cancer has successfully invaded the body and taken a beachhead. Malignant tumors have the ability to metastasize (spread to other parts of the body), disrupt the normal function of the body, and assault other tissues.

Different types of cancer behave differently in the body. Lung cancer and breast cancer, to name two of the most common, grow at different rates and respond to different treatments, which is why cancer treatments have become more specialized in the last twenty years. No matter what cancer is present in the body, however, you can be sure that cancer cells *will* travel to other parts of the body. Just remember that doctors always name the type of cancer from where it *began,* not where it has spread. For example, cancer that begins in the lungs before spreading to the liver will always be known as lung cancer.

INHIBIT VS. PROMOTE

Since cancer, by definition, occurs when damaged cells assault the body, researchers have determined that some factors *inhibit* or *promote* the growth of cancer in the body. Examples of *inhibitors* would be nutrients found in fruits and vegetables, as well as certain vitamins. Drinking plenty of water allows the kidneys and liver to operate at full capacity and flush waste and toxins out of the body's digestive and urinary tracts, which is where cancer cells tend to congregate. You hear about cancer of the colon, prostate, liver, and stomach; you don't hear about cancer of the elbow or knee.

On the other hand, examples of *promoters* would be smoking cigarettes or eating a diet of fried foods rich in trans-fatty acids or coming into contact with cancer-causing substances, also known as carcinogens. Tobacco smoke, pesticides, air pollution, and industrial chemicals (such as asbestos) can trigger the initiation of cancer, which can take years to develop into a mass and many more years to detect, as was the case with Grandma Rose.

While environmental elements behind cancer are significant, at the end of the day, lifestyle factors are the main causes of cancer. Yes, genetics and family history do play a role (between 5 and 10 percent of all cancers are clearly hereditary), but the choices in the food we eat, the amount of time we exercise, the hygiene we practice, the stress we undergo, and the otherwise imbalanced lives we lead account for about 65 percent of cancer deaths in the United States, according to the Harvard University School of Public Health.[5]

A breakdown of the 570,000 deaths annually looks like this:

Poor diet and obesity	30 percent
Smoking	30 percent
Genetics	10 percent
Carcinogens in the workplace	5 percent
Family history	5 percent
Lack of exercise	5 percent
Viruses	5 percent
Alcohol	3 percent
Reproductive factors	3 percent
Socioeconomic status	3 percent
Environmental pollution	2 percent[6]

Review this list one more time. Did you notice that eating the wrong foods and gaining too much weight—"poor diet and obesity"—rank just as high as smoking for causing cancer deaths? I would have thought that smoking would be a runaway winner in the cancer sweepstakes, but this breakdown is stark evidence that *what we eat* can be just as damaging as *what we do*.

CONVENTIONAL TREATMENT OPTIONS

The question on anyone's mind after receiving the confirmation of a cancer diagnosis is *What will I do to treat this disease?* This can be a life-or-death decision because cancer patients often do not have the luxury of traveling down certain treatment avenues before deciding on another approach. On most occasions, it's a race against time. While cancer is a systematic disease that steadily marches forward, treatment is not one-size-fits-all. You should choose a treatment plan that reaches you on a number of levels, including physical, mental, emotional, and spiritual.

The vast majority of cancer patients turn to conventional medicine for several reasons:

- Medically speaking, that's where they started, by seeing an oncologist to determine what kind of cancer they had and what stage it was.

- The conventional medical world feels comfortable to them because that is what they know.

- They are not used to thinking about outside-the-box alternative treatments.

- Their insurance plan covers only conventional treatments.

The conventional medicine route follows four basic options:

1. *Surgery.* Growing up as the son of a naturopathic doctor and chiropractor, I heard my father and mother express their distrust of "knife-happy" surgeons ready to cut first, then seek other approaches later. There's evidence that even a simple biopsy can cause cancer to spread. Having said that, I understand that there are times when surgery is not only prudent or necessary, but often the correct therapeutic approach to take. A skilled surgeon can wield a razor-sharp scalpel to scrape, slice, and sliver malignant growths of cancer.

Cutting out and removing tumorous tissues is the oldest known form of conventional cancer treatment. Thanks to improved surgical techniques and laparoscopic technology, surgery is far less invasive than it was a decade or two ago. Most people with cancer submit to some sort of surgery, according to the American Cancer Society.

2. *Radiation.* Radioactive waves or a stream of particles is used to alter the genetic code of cancerous cells inside the body. Side effects are fatigue, skin damage, loss of brain function, and damage to local tissues. About half of all people with cancer will receive radiation during their cancer treatment.

3. *Chemotherapy.* The definition of chemotherapy is taking medicines, or drugs, to treat cancer. Patients receiving chemotherapy treatment (usually directly into a vein through intravenous transfusions) often experience nausea, hair loss, fatigue, and sores inside the mouth.

4. *Immunotherapy.* The newest weapon that cancer specialists have at their disposal is immunotherapy, which is using certain parts of the immune system to fight the cancer cells inside the body. This is accomplished by stimulating the immune system to work harder against the damaged cells inside the body.

While conventional therapies have been proven to drive cancer into remission, patients and families sometimes hear their doctors talk about "investigational treatment," which means the treatment protocol is part of a clinical trial to determine whether it is a safe and effective way to treat cancer.

ALTERNATIVE CANCER TREATMENTS

Alternative therapies for cancer have not been proven to cure cancer, but sometimes—and I mean sometimes—alternative medicine has effectively treated the disease by using a holistic approach that treats the whole body rather than the area of the body with cancer. Alternative medicine practitioners believe that the cancer developed, for the most part, from a problem in the body's immune system or some other kind of imbalance in the body—an imbalance created from improper lifestyle habits and poor nutrition, coupled with an overabundance of stored toxins.

The list of alternative cancer therapies is much longer, which is not an indictment of the medical profession but an acknowledgment that when people are facing a life-and-death struggle, they are willing to try anything to stay alive. Most often, those fighting cancer to the bitter end complement their conventional treatments with an alternative approach.

Alternative treatments usually involve mind-body therapies, herbal therapies, nutritional therapies, and metabolic therapies. They range from colon cleansing to coffee enemas, from drinking essiac tea to injecting specially processed animal embryo tissue into the body. Hypnosis, biofeedback, and psychological counseling focus on the role of emotions in fighting the disease.

One alternative medical approach has been the use of laetrile, a synthetic form of a chemical found in apricot pits, apple seeds, and bitter almonds.[7] Cancer patients such as Hollywood actor Steve McQueen traveled to Mexico to receive laetrile shots, but laetrile treatment has never stood up to medical scrutiny. The National Cancer Institute conducted two studies of laetrile in the early 1980s, under the auspices of the Mayo Clinic, and the results were clear-cut: not one patient was cured or stabilized.[8]

Many patients realize that supplementing their conventional cancer care with alternative medicine may or may not work, but when it's your life on the line, the will to live has a way of searching for every option.

A Road Map from Here

The Great Physician's Rx for Cancer is not guaranteed to prevent or treat cancer, and I would never want anyone to represent this book as promising a "cure" for this deadly disease. I second the disclaimer at the beginning of this book.

What I'm hoping is that *The Great Physician's Rx for Cancer* will do one of two things:

1. Give you the best possible chance never to develop cancer.

2. Augment whatever therapy—conventional or alternative—you're seeking to treat your cancer and live a long, healthy life.

My approach is based on seven keys to unlock the body's healthy potential that were established in my foundational book *The Great Physician's Rx for Health and Wellness:*

- Key #1: Eat to live.

- Key #2: Supplement your diet with whole food nutritionals, living nutrients, and superfoods.

- Key #3: Practice advanced hygiene.

- Key #4: Condition your body with exercise and body therapies.

- Key #5: Reduce toxins in your environment.

- Key #6: Avoid deadly emotions.

- Key #7: Live a life of prayer and purpose.

Each of these keys should directly support your desire to prevent or triumph over cancer, and I believe each and every one of us has a God-given health potential that can be unlocked only with the right keys. I'm asking you to incorporate these timeless principles and allow the living God to transform your health as you honor Him physically, mentally, emotionally, and spiritually.

KEY #1

Eat to Live

The first key that I present in *The Great Physician's Rx for Cancer* happens to be the most important. According to the National Academy of Sciences, 60 percent of all cancers in women and 40 percent of all cancers in men can be linked to dietary and nutritional factors.[1] In other words, what you eat could prevent cancer or, if you've been diagnosed with this disease, help you achieve victory.

How do you "eat to live" when it comes to cancer? By following these two foundational principles:

1. Eat what God created for food.
2. Eat food in a form that is healthy for the body.

I'll get into specifics shortly, but since cancer usually signifies a problem with the immune system or an imbalance inside the body, eating foods that God created and are grown, raised, produced, and prepared healthfully is a strong prescription for reducing the ability of cancerous cells to grow inside your body. Eating foods that God created in a form that is healthy for the body means choosing foods as close to the natural source as possible, which will nourish your body, help you perform at optimal levels, and give you the healthiest life possible. As you can probably figure out by now, I'm a proponent of natural foods grown organically.

What About Eating and Cancer Treatment?

If you're undergoing cancer treatment, you probably don't feel like eating *anything*. I can't speak from experience since I've never undergone chemotherapy or radiation treatment.

Cancer treatment, with its attendant side effects, is brutal on the body because radiation and chemotherapy kill cancer cells *and* healthy living cells. Technological advances have eased the unpleasant discomfort, but a day of cancer treatment is no day at the beach. Patients often complain of a poor appetite or the side effects of treatment: nausea, vomiting, or mouth sores. Foods taste different, and it's difficult to summon the energy to bring the fork to your mouth.

You have to eat, however, because every bite you take can be just as important as the treatments you're enduring. Bodies fueled with foods high in carbohydrates (pastries, sweets, and ice cream) don't have the nutritional gravitas to rebuild damaged tissues, fight infection, or cope with the side effects of treatment.

Often during treatment, people will seek out comfort foods, wistfully hoping that meat loaf smothered in gravy or barbecued pork dripping with sweet sauce will lift their spirits and renew their desire to fight to the finish. While I'm sympathetic, I know with all of my heart that when Grandma Rose stopped eating healthy, she opened the door for cancer to return. When you're undergoing chemotherapy and other conventional cancer treatments, it's best to consume easily digestible foods and beverages such as cultured dairy products (yogurt and kefir) mixed with honey and fruit and flaxseed oil. Fresh fruits, vegetable juices, and protein foods such as soft-boiled eggs or baked or steamed fish are also recommended.

This is also a great time to introduce whole food nutritional supplements to your diet, which you'll learn about in the next chapter.

For the cancer patient, optimizing nutrition begins with an awareness of what you are sending to your digestive tract. To begin with, everything you put into your mouth is a protein, a fat, or a carbohydrate. Following correct dietary principles will be key because each of these nutrients positively or negatively affects your body's cells, which are the foundation of life.

Let's take a closer look at these macronutrients.

THE FIRST WORD ON PROTEINS

Proteins, one of the basic components of foods, are the essential building blocks of the body, and they are involved in the function of every living cell. One of protein's main tasks is to provide specific nutrient material to grow and repair cells—even cancerous ones.

All proteins are combinations of twenty-two amino acids, which build body organs, muscles, and nerves, to name a few important duties. Your body, however, cannot produce all twenty-two amino acids that you need to live a robust life. Scientists have discovered that eight essential amino acids are missing, meaning that they must come from other sources outside the body. I know the following fact drives vegetarians and vegans crazy, but animal protein—chicken, beef, lamb, dairy, eggs, and so on—is the *only* complete protein source providing the Big Eight amino acids.

I don't believe that the best and most healthy sources of animal protein come from your supermarket's meat case. Commercially raised livestock, fish, and poultry are routinely fed grain and meal laced with hormones, nitrates, and pesticides—chemicals that have been investigated as possible carcinogenic substances. In this country, cattle routinely chew on feedstuffs with hormones (melengestrol acetate, or MGA, improves the growth rate in feedlot heifers) and buffers (sodium bicarbonate works on acidity in the digestive tract that is caused from the animal's diet and other unhealthy substances consumed). These additives help livestock owners fatten up their herd, which fattens their bottom lines, but these practices may pose health risks to humans who dine on this meat.

The best approach for a cancer patient is to eat the healthiest sources of animal protein available, which come from organically raised cattle, sheep, goats, buffalo, and venison—animals that graze on pastureland grasses. Grass-fed beef is leaner and lower in calories than grain-fed beef.

The same goes for free-range chicken, which is the antithesis of modern methods of chicken production. These days, commercially raised chickens are raised in long, windowless sheds, cooped up without fresh air, and fed from hoppers dispensing food pellets and water. These chickens live miserable lives until they're plump enough to slaughter, as compared to their country cousins, who are allowed to roam around and hunt and peck for their food.

I'm also a huge fan of eating fish captured from lakes, streambeds, or ocean depths. Fish with scales and fins caught in the wild are lean sources of protein and provide all the essential amino acids. Wild fish, which is nutritionally far superior to farm-raised, should be consumed liberally.

ROUNDTABLE ON FATS

God, in His infinite wisdom, created fats as a concentrated source of energy and source material for cell membranes and various hormones. Healthy fats have a protective effect against heart disease, play a vital role in the health of our bones, enhance the immune system, protect the liver from alcohol and other toxins, and guard against harmful microorganisms in the digestive tract, where 20 percent of new cancer cases originate. Fats add taste to food and provide satiety; otherwise, we would be raiding the refrigerator within an hour if fats didn't give us that full feeling.

The right kinds of fats can protect us from cancer. The problem with the standard American diet is that people eat too many of the wrong foods containing the wrong fats and not enough of the right foods with the right fats. "Wrong fats" are hydrogenated oils containing trans fats, which raise LDL cholesterol rates, clog arteries, cause heart attacks, and also increase the incidence of most cancers.

As for the "right fats," I'm referring to foods loaded with omega-3 polyunsaturated fats, monounsaturated (omega-9) fatty acids, and conjugated linoleic acid (CLA), as well as healthy saturated fats containing short- and medium-chain fatty acids, such as butter and coconut oil. These good fats are found in a wide range of foods including salmon, lamb, and goat meat; in dairy products derived from goat's milk, sheep's milk, and cow's milk from grass-fed animals; and in flaxseeds, walnuts, olives, macadamia nuts, and avocados. Eating too many of the wrong fats—which are usually found in highly processed foods containing partially hydrogenated oils—has become a well-known cancer risk.

Many of our processed foods—foods that God definitely did *not* create—contain trans fats. Food conglomerates that produce plastic-wrapped snack foods use hydrogenated oil in the manufacturing process. Hydrogenated oils are liquid fats that have been injected with hydrogen gas at high temperatures under high pressure to make them solid at room temperature. Why do food producers employ so much chemistry? Because it allows them to produce a more competitively priced product with a longer shelf life that behaves like . . . well, a saturated fat.

My advice is to stay away from packaged dessert treats and store aisles stuffed with processed foods and eat as many foods in their natural state as possible. Eat a couple of organic eggs in the morning. Fill your lunch plate with organic lettuce, tomatoes, and carrots. Snack on raw fruit between meals. At dinnertime, eat a balanced meal of organically produced beef, a more exotic grain like quinoa, and vegetables in season. When cooking, use butter or extra virgin coconut oil. All of the aforementioned foods are loaded with vitamins, antioxidants, fiber, omega-3 fatty acids, and many other micronutrients that play a crucial role in the body's fight against cancer.

You should make good fats a part of your daily diet. Dr. Johanna Budwig, a German biochemist, made this argument as far back as the 1950s when she suggested mixing flaxseed oil with quark or cottage cheese. She argued that the unsaturated high omega-3 fats in flaxseed oil, combined with the sulfur proteins of quark or cottage cheese, gave the body's cells the vital energy needed to fight cancer.[2]

WINNING CARBOHYDRATES

By definition, carbohydrates are the starches and sugars produced by plant foods, and they are carried in the blood as glucose and regulated by insulin, a hormone that holds the key to the body cell's nutritional door. Thanks to the low-carb diet popularized by Dr. Robert Atkins, Americans have been on a carbohydrate witch hunt for the last five or ten years. The premise behind these trendy books is that burning excess carbohydrates at the stake, so to speak, is the panacea for weight loss.

The Atkins diet, to single out the oldest and most widely practiced low-carb diet, calls for a high consumption of conventionally raised and processed meats (ham, bacon, pepperoni, salami, and hot dogs) that are high in unhealthy fats, which in my mind only *increases* your cancer risk since their curing process introduces additives like nitrates, which can convert to nitrite, which can form into nitrosamines, a powerful cancer-causing chemical. The Atkins diet also forbids plentiful amounts of fruits and vegetables.

So I have a question: How does one reconcile that nutritional advice with the National Cancer Institute recommendation that we eat at least five servings of fruits and vegetables daily to significantly reduce the risk of developing cancer? I'm not going out on a limb when I note that you will always be better off eating fruits and vegetables rather than incorporating bacon strips and salami wedges into your meals.

Returning to our discussion about carbohydrates, there is an old saying that sounds more like an old wives' tale, but it's worth discussing: "Sugar feeds cancer." This saying dates back seventy-five years when German biochemist and medical doctor Otto Warburg captured the Nobel Prize in 1931 for demonstrating that cancer cells have a different energy metabolism when compared to healthy cells.

If you're saying to yourself, *So what?* let me try to explain. The science behind this catchphrase goes like this: when you eat large amounts of sugar or starches, the body experiences a spike in blood sugar levels. When blood sugar levels rise, two things happen:

1. The body releases insulin to control the spike in blood sugar levels.

2. Immunity levels are depressed to some degree, which makes you more vulnerable to viral or bacterial infections.

Cancer cells are anaerobic, meaning that they don't need oxygen to derive their energy. Instead, they use carbon dioxide. Many bacteria live the same way. If you inject the bacteria that cause tetanus into laboratory mice with cancer, then the bacteria will live and give the mice tetanus; if you inject the same bacteria into healthy mice with no cancer, they will not develop tetanus. This happens because every place in the body of a healthy mouse has oxygen.

In the world of cancer, researchers now agree that a patient's high blood sugar level feeds cancerous tumors. They've noticed how malignant tumors usually exhibit an increase in anaerobic glycolysis, which is a two-buck description of a process in which cancer cells use glucose as a fuel. Doctors rely on this knowledge when they administer a positron-emission tomography, or PET, scan.

Glucose is the main form of sugar that the body utilizes for energy production. Other sugars, like fructose in food, are converted by the liver into glucose for the body to use. After the liver takes care of these sugars, it releases them slowly into the bloodstream so that the blood sugar will stay under control. We use the glycemic index to measure how a given food affects blood glucose levels.

A high-sugar diet has always been unhealthy, but follow-up research on Dr. Warburg's findings confirms what I feel in my gut: eating sugary foods while fighting cancer lessens your odds for survival. Nancy Appleton, Ph.D., listed seventy-six ways that sugar can ruin you even if you're in the peak of health, but it was the first one that caught my eye: sugar can suppress your immune system and impair your defenses against infectious disease.[3]

I'm not talking about eliminating all sugar from your diet, because doing so would also mean doing away with God-created foods that contain natural sugars—fruits, vegetables, yogurt, and honey. In fact, Croatian researchers at the University of Zagreb say that eating honey and other bee products may prevent cancer or slow it down, based on tests with laboratory mice.[4]

But completely removing any *refined* sugar, which is found in just about every processed food known to man, from store-bought cookies to ketchup, from peanut butter to raspberry jam, from bread to pasta, from colas to sweet teas, is a definite plus for the body. Always eat a balance of the best carbohydrates with the best proteins and fats at every meal to balance your blood sugar.

Here's how the medical establishment behind WebMD sums up the "sugar and cancer" topic:

Cancer cells in a tumor like to eat glucose and will alter the metabolism of the body to get more. They do this by increasing liver gluconeogenesis from amino acids, which leads to a loss of muscle tissue from the skeleton and internal organs. Insulin resistance is increased so that glucose will not be as able to enter healthy cells. All of this results in hyperglycemia, or high blood sugar levels.

One of the purposes of nutrition therapy for cancer is to deny the growing tumor glucose while providing enough for the central nervous system and red blood cell formation. This can be done in a crude way by keeping the blood sugar levels even. You can do this by following these guidelines:

- Avoiding eating or drinking *anything* that tastes sweet on an empty stomach. This includes sweet-tasting fruit and vegetable juices, fruit, soda pop, sweetened refined cereals, honey, or any liquid sweetened with any form of sugar.

- Always eat a balanced meal with mixed foods. A meal rich in complex carbohydrates and fiber will slow the release of food from the stomach, thereby slowing the release of glucose from the meal.

- Eat sweet whole foods such as fruit only with meals. Drink diluted low-sugar fruit and vegetable juices only with fat-containing meals.

  A diet in which most of the calories came from unrefined carbohydrates is also rich in many other nutrients that can inhibit the growth of cancer cells.[5]

Apart from potatoes and corn, unrefined carbohydrates are grains such as wheat, rye, rice, and barley. Unrefined carbohydrates still contain the whole grain, including the bran and the germ, so they're higher in fiber and healthy fatty acids. The staple of most diets around the world—wheat—is hard to find in an unrefined state because nearly all wheat is subjected to an "enriching" process.

Since most Americans eat foods with refined white flour for every meal, however, be aware that any excess refined carbohydrates in the blood system feed normal cells as well as cancerous cells. The key is to boost your immune system—and fight the cancerous cells—by not giving them the nutrients necessary for growth. Instead, look for carbohydrate foods that are *unrefined,* and the best sources are fruits and vegetables, sprouted grains, cultured dairy, honey, nuts, seeds, and legumes—preferably organic and consumed raw, if possible. It's better to buy organic flour with the words *stone ground, yeast free,* or *sprouted* on the package label.

NUTRITION RECOMMENDATIONS

Most doctors and nurses will say that recommendations about food and eating for cancer patients can be different from the usual suggestions for healthy eating. They will stress eating lots of fruits, vegetables, and whole grain breads and cereals, consuming moderate amounts of meat and dairy products, and cutting back on sugar and fats.

I don't think it should take a cancer diagnosis to shake up what one chooses to eat. Much of what conventional medicine recommends for cancer patients is part of the Great Physician's Rx for health and wellness, but I want to make additional points in this section, as well as list my top healing foods. Let's take a closer look at what we eat.

1. Meats

There's cause for concern regarding meat, especially red meat, since several scientific studies describe a relationship between cancer and red meat consumption. One of the latest, a study of 500,000 men and women from ten European countries, showed that people who ate the most red meat and processed meat (hot dogs, sausages, and salami) had a higher risk of colon cancer.[6]

Food processing companies churning out breakfast links, bacon, lunch meats, hot dogs, bratwurst, and other sausages use preservatives called nitrates to give meats their blood-red color, convey flavor, and resist the development of botulism spores. Nitrates, as mentioned earlier, can covert to nitrites, and nitrites have been studied for decades in public and private settings and found to cause cancer and tumors in test animals. Food producers, however, point to a National Academy of Sciences review indicating that nitrites do not directly act as a carcinogen in animals and that nitrates, when converted to nitrites in the human body, are not carcinogenic.[7] Since this landmark study happened in 1981, the argument of whether nitrites are carcinogenic has been going on for twenty-five years. I feel that if you don't eat these processed meats in the first place, then the question of whether nitrites are carcinogenic becomes moot.

I have other reasons for recommending that you stay away from bacon and ham lunch meat. In all of my previous books, I've consistently pointed out that pork—America's "other white meat"—should be avoided because pigs were called "unclean" in Leviticus and Deuteronomy. God, in His infinite wisdom, created pigs as scavengers—animals that survive just fine on any farm slop or water swill tossed their way. Pigs have a simple stomach arrangement: whatever a pig eats goes down the hatch, straight into the stomach, and out the back door in four hours max. They'll even eat their own excrement, if hungry enough.

Even if you decide to keep eating commercial beef instead of the organic version, I absolutely urge you to stop eating pork. Read Leviticus 11 and Deuteronomy 14 to learn what God said about eating clean versus unclean animals, where Hebrew words used to describe unclean meats can be translated as "foul" and "putrid," the same terms that describe human waste.

Meanwhile, other studies show that young women who eat a lot of red meat—basically a hamburger diet—increase their risk of breast cancer, or double that risk according to another study.[8] Men are more susceptible to developing prostate cancer or pancreatic cancer with a diet high in red meats.

These studies usually don't say *why* there's a link between red meat and cancer; all they note is the scientific link between the two. My gut says that hormones, pesticides, and herbicides taint our commercial meat supply, and that meat eaters are likely consuming biblically "unclean" processed and cured meats. I would like to see a study done of a possible link between cancer and the best sources of meat—organically raised cattle, buffalo, lamb, and venison that graze on nature's bountiful grasses. I still believe that eating this source of animal protein—in the right amounts—will always be healthy for you.

The healthiest meat of all is fish, and in the European study I quoted earlier, those who consumed the most fish had the *lowest* risk of colon cancer. As far as a meat source is concerned, fish caught in the wild are one of the top healing foods that I mention in this chapter. Wild-caught fish are a rich source of omega-3 fatty acids, which may help prevent prostate cancer, according to a large study of Swedish men. These fatty acids, along with selenium, prevent the oxidation of cells in the progression of cancer. The antioxidant qualities in fish such as herring, mackerel, and salmon are recommended. You can purchase fresh salmon and other wild-caught fish from your local fish market or health food store.

2. Dairy Products

Medical doctors lump the saturated fats in dairy products with red meat, implicating the fat intake as a key factor behind higher cancer rates. Thus, doctors recommend that we should eat full-fat dairy products in moderation, and when we do reach for a half-gallon of milk, we should be sure to choose a low-fat version such as 2 percent or skim milk.

I don't see things the same way because drinking 2 percent or skim milk makes the milk less nutritious and less digestible, and can cause allergies. When it comes to preventing cancer, dairy products derived from goat's milk and sheep's milk are healthier than those from cows, although dairy products from organic or grass-fed cows can be excellent as well. Why are goat's milk and goat's cheese so much better for you? The difference lies in the goat milk's structure: its fat and protein molecules are tiny in size, which allows for rapid absorption in the digestive tract. Goat's milk is less allergenic because it does not contain the same complex proteins found in cow's milk. Cultured dairy, such as yogurt and kefir, provides an excellent source of easily digestible protein, B vitamins, calcium, and probiotics, as well as other cancer-fighting compounds such as L-lactic acid.

3. Fruits and Vegetables (and their juices)

This has to be the biggest no-brainer. Everyone involved with cancer, from the top medical specialists to those promoting alternative cures, sings from the same song sheet: you need to increase your fruit and veggie consumption to prevent or battle cancer. Yet the average American consumes far less than the recommended five to nine servings of fruits and vegetables daily, which are some of the most beneficial cancer-preventing foods that God created on this planet.

Fruits and vegetables right from the fields are the nutritional antithesis of processed foods, which come off an assembly line at a factory or industrial bakery. Fruits and veggies contain compounds that work to detoxify carcinogens. Plant foods are the best sources in nature for antioxidants, which neutralize toxic substances in the body known as free radicals. Some of these cancer-fighting antioxidants are vitamin A, beta-carotene, lycopene, vitamin C (known as a nitrate scavenger), vitamin E (which protects cell membranes and goes after free radicals as well), and selenium, which I mentioned earlier for its antioxidant properties.

Many fruit and vegetable foods contain immune-boosting and cancer-fighting chemicals; Asian mushrooms (shiitake, maitake, and reishi), berries (blueberries and raspberries), and other fruits (pomegranates and grapes) are only a few examples. Pomegranate juice showed promise against prostate cancer in research conducted at the University of Wisconsin and released in 2005. Human prostate cancer cells were injected into laboratory mice, which were then fed a pomegranate extract. Tumor growth was significantly inhibited, and survival was prolonged.[9] Researchers noted that pomegranate juice is higher in antioxidant activity than red wine and green tea.

You should eat a minimum of two or three fresh fruits daily. They make excellent snacks. As for vegetables, try to eat four to six servings a day, with a fresh, raw salad included in the mix. A typical serving is one-half cup.

I'm also a big fan of consuming raw fruit and vegetable juices as a concentrated source of vitamins, minerals, and antioxidants. Max Gerson, M.D., a German-born physician who lived from 1881 to 1959, employed a therapy of raw vegetable and fruit juicing, combined with selected additional foods, to treat cancer. Dr. Gerson believed the body's metabolism worked most effectively when the diet consisted of alkalizing foods such as raw vegetable and fruit juices, which help maintain the body's pH and eliminate toxins that hinder cellular function.

Potassium also plays a role in maintaining cellular pH. When potassium moves into or out of the cell, it is exchanged with hydrogen, which plays a vital role in pH cellular balance. One of the best ways to increase alkalinity in the diet is to increase levels of the alkalizing mineral potassium and decrease sodium. This can be accomplished by consuming liberal amounts of fresh vegetable and fruit juices. Some of the foods highest in potassium are apricots, figs, carrots, and greens such as spinach, but most fruits and veggies are good sources of potassium. Other alkalizing compounds include apple cider vinegar and fresh lemon juice.

4. Soaked and Sprouted Seeds and Grains

Like fruits and vegetables, whole grains, seeds, nuts, and breads made with sprouted or sour-leavened grains are linked to studies suggesting that eating them reduces some kinds of cancers. Apparently the fiber, vitamins, phytochemicals, and antioxidants in properly prepared whole grains—wheat, corn, oats, and rice—appear to work together in the fight against this deadly disease. *Whole grain* means the bran and germ are left on the grain during processing. *Soaked and sprouted grains* retain their plant enzymes when they are not cooked.

As for your new cancer-friendly diet, say good-bye to white bread, hello to sprouted or sour-leavened whole wheat, rye, or flaxseed breads. Say good-bye to white rice, hello to brown rice and other healthy grains such as amaranth, quinoa, millet, and buckwheat. Say good-bye to pasta made from white enriched flour, hello to sprouted grain or spelt pasta, quinoa, barley, or couscous.

5. Cultured and Fermented Vegetables

Often greeted with upturned noses at the dinner table, fermented vegetables such as sauerkraut, pickled carrots, beets, or cucumbers help reestablish the natural balance of the digestive system. Fermented vegetables like sauerkraut are brimming with vitamins, such as vitamin C, and contain almost four times the cancer-fighting nutrients as unfermented cabbage.

If you've never put a fork on any of these foods before, I urge you to sample sauerkraut or pickled beets, which are readily available in health food stores.

6. Teas and Spices

Research suggests that the antioxidants in green tea shut down a key molecule that can play a significant role in the development of cancer.[10] This key molecule is known as the aryl hydrocarbon (AH) receptor, which has the ability to trigger potentially harmful gene activity. Researchers are finding that antioxidant chemicals in other types of tea, including white and oolong, enhance the health of the body by inactivating potentially carcinogenic free radicals. Two chemicals present in green tea inhibit AH activity, so you may want to think about switching your favorite hot drink to green, white, or oolong tea.

A household spice in your cupboard may have cancer-fighting properties. Turmeric, a spice used in curry dishes that contains a compound called curcumin, has inhibited the growth of melanoma cells as well as breast and pancreatic cancers.[11] Turmeric is rich in plant compounds that are proving to be potent anti-tumor agents. Currently the University of Michigan Medical School is conducting a national trial to determine if another household spice—ginger—controls nausea and vomiting in cancer patients receiving chemotherapy treatment. Ginger, and other plants in its genus group, contains chemicals that have also been shown to prevent cancer.[12]

7. Water

Water isn't a food, of course, but this calorie-free and sugar-free substance performs many vital tasks for the body: regulating the body temperature, carrying nutrients and oxygen to the cells, cushioning joints, protecting organs and tissues, and removing toxins. Water happens to be the perfect fluid replacement; only God could come up with a liquid that makes up 92 percent of your blood plasma and 50 percent of everything else in your body.

Earlier in this chapter, I mentioned how cancer cells are somewhat anaerobic, meaning they do not like oxygen. Well, water brings oxygen to cancer cells through the bloodstream; the more well hydrated your body is, the better your body can prevent or fight cancer. "I am convinced that water is the best naturally preventive, and *curative,* cancer medication in the world," said F. Batmanghelidj, M.D., author of *You're Not Sick, You're Thirsty!* Dr. Batmanghelidj says that dehydration causes a drastic system disturbance in the physiology of the body and causes disruptions that ultimately allow for cancer formation and the invasive growth of new tissue.[13]

You should drink a minimum of eight glasses of water a day to stay hydrated. Drinking plenty of water is not only healthy for the body, but it may save your life.

What Not to Eat

Whether you're trying to avoid cancer in the future, or you're in the fight of your life against this disease, here is a list of foods that should never find a way onto your plate or into your hands. I call them the Dirty Dozen. Some I've already discussed elsewhere in this chapter, while the rest are presented here with a short commentary:

1. *Processed meat and pork products.* These meats top my list because they are staples in the standard American diet and are extremely unhealthy.

2. *Shellfish and fish without fins and scales, such as catfish, shark, and eel.* Am I saying au revoir, sayonara, and adios to lobster thermidor, shrimp tempura, and carnitas burritos? That's what I'm saying.

3. *Hydrogenated oils.* Margarine and shortening are taboo, as well as any commercial cakes, pastries, desserts, and anything with the words *hydrogenated* or *partially hydrogenated* on the label.

4. *Artificial sweeteners.* Aspartame (found in NutraSweet and Equal), saccharin (Sweet 'N Low), and sucralose (Splenda) are chemicals several hundred times sweeter than sugar. Do they cause cancer? Hard to say. The Food and Drug Administration says that you would have to drink fifteen diet sodas or consume eighty-five packets of Equal each day to cross a certain threshold. At one time, diet drinks and sugar-free gum with saccharin came with the warning label—"Use of this product may be hazardous to your health"—but the FDA took saccharin off the list of known carcinogens in 2000. In my book, however, artificial sweeteners should be completely avoided.

5. *White flour.* White flour isn't a problematic chemical like artificial sweeteners, but it's virtually worthless and not healthy for you.

6. *White sugar.* "Sugar feeds cancer," right? Enough said.

7. *Soft drinks.* They are nothing more than liquefied sugar. A twenty-ounce can of Coke or Pepsi is the equivalent of eating fifteen teaspoons of sugar. Popular soft drinks also contain chemicals that cause the body to become more acidic, which is not a great Rx for cancer.

8. *Corn syrup.* This is just another version of sugar and just as dangerous for cancer patients.

9. *Pasteurized homogenized skim milk.* Like I said, whole organic, nonhomogenized milk is better, and goat's milk is best.

10. *Hydrolyzed soy protein.* Hydrolyzed soy protein is found in imitation meat products such as imitation crab. I would look at hydrolyzed soy protein as I would regard meat cured with nitrites: stay away from it. You're always going to be better off eating organic meats.

11. *Artificial flavors and colors.* These are never good for you under the best of circumstances, and certainly not when you're battling cancer.

12. *Excessive alcohol.* Although studies point out the benefits of drinking small amounts of red wine for the heart (part of the "French Paradox"), the fact remains that alcohol contains lots of calories, and wine usually contains lots of sugar—and sugar feeds cancer. A precursor to liver cancer is cirrhosis of the liver, which stems from alcoholism and binge drinking. And here's a sobering statement: the National Institute on Alcohol Abuse and Alcoholism says that there is considerable evidence linking heavy alcohol consumption and increased risk for cancer, with an estimated 2 to 4 percent of all cancer cases thought to be caused directly or indirectly by alcohol.[14]

EAT: What Foods Are Extraordinary, Average, or Trouble?

I've prepared a comprehensive list of foods that are ranked in descending order based on their health-giving qualities. Foods at the top of the list are healthier than those at the bottom. The best foods to serve and eat are what I call extraordinary, which God created for us to eat and will give you the best chance not to develop cancer. If you are battling cancer, however, it is best to consume foods from the Extraordinary category more than 75 percent of the time.

Foods in the Average category should make up less than 25 percent of your daily diet. If you're in the throes of a cancer battle, consume these foods sparingly.

Foods in the Trouble category should be consumed with extreme caution. If you are dealing with a cancer diagnosis or seek to give your body the best chance to fight off cancer, you should avoid these foods completely.

For a complete listing of Extraordinary, Average, and Trouble Foods, visit www.BiblicalHealthInstitute.com/EAT.

To Fast or Not to Fast?

In *The Great Physician's Rx for Health and Wellness*, I recommend a partial one-day fast each week for its physical as well as spiritual benefits. It's amazing what God will show you when you give up sustenance for Him.

Fasting on only water is problematic, however, if your body is weakened by chemotherapy or radiation treatment for cancer. When you're fighting for your life, you need to gird your strength for treatment.

While that's true, a fast gives your body a needed break from the digestive process, which frees up the metabolic enzymes to cleanse the body and break down the residual waste material stored in your body. A juice fast can accomplish this goal while giving the body a small amount of needed calories and helping alkalize the body. I recommend a three-day juice fast by drinking eight twelve-ounce glasses of raw juices mixed with either digestive enzymes or green superfoods in the following format:

- From waking until 2:00 p.m., drink four eight- to twelve-ounce drinks of carrot/apple juice made in a home juicer with one tablespoon or ten capsules of plant-based digestive enzyme powder (for recommended brands, visit www.BiblicalHealthInstitute.com and click on the GPRx Resource Guide).

- From 2:00 p.m. until bedtime, drink four eight- to twelve-ounce drinks of carrot/celery/parsley blended in a juicer with one tablespoon of a green superfood powder or five green superfood caplets (for recommended products, visit www.BiblicalHealth Institute.com and click on the GPRx Resource Guide).

After three days of this juice fast, I recommend eating extremely healthy foods for four days. (See the Great Physician's Rx for Cancer Battle Plan on page 73 for more information.)

℞ THE GREAT PHYSICIAN'S Rx FOR CANCER: EAT TO LIVE

- *Eat only foods God created.*

- *Eat foods in a form that is healthy for the body.*

- *Avoid foods with sugar.*

- *Increase consumption of raw fruits and vegetables.*

- *Go on periodic vegetable and fruit juice fasts using fresh juices.*

Take Action

To learn how to incorporate the principles of eating to live into your daily life, please turn to page 73 for the Great Physician's Rx for Cancer Battle Plan.

KEY #2

Supplement Your Diet with Whole Food Nutritionals, Living Nutrients, and Superfoods

If you ask a doctor whether taking multivitamins and nutritional supplements is important in the prevention of or treatment for cancer, he will probably reply that a balanced diet is central, that no diet or nutritional plan can "cure" cancer, and that taking vitamin or mineral supplements should never be considered a substitute for medical care. And last but not least, you shouldn't take any supplements without a doctor's knowledge and consent.

That cautious answer is a form of defensive medicine that doesn't recognize the enormous potential of—and evidence for—various nutritional supplements. Taking multivitamins and supplements can do more than cover your bases: they can keep you in the game against cancer—and perhaps help you beat it.

When Grandma Rose asked me for help, she wasn't a big vitamin taker. Popping a couple of vitamin C tablets down the hatch each morning was about it. As part of my research studying naturopathic medicine and nutrition, I studied the body's immune system and how it related to cancer. My grandma needed to "activate" her immune cells to fight off the cancer cells. Certain compounds, including edible fungi, stimulated the activation of immune cells through the production of cytokines, which are immune cell secretions that facilitate cell-to-cell communication.

In other words, these "good" cytokines could tell the "bad" cancer cells to go jump off a cliff, metaphorically speaking.

Here's the regimen I suggested for Grandma Rose to take:

- a whole food multivitamin

- a green superfood

- a probiotic containing SBOs (soil-based organisms)

- large amounts of plant-based enzymes

- goat's milk protein powder

- a whole food fiber blend

- an immune-enhancing mushroom formula

The last item was a prototype supplement that I was developing. This supplement contained ten different mushrooms, as well as aloe vera and cat's claw fermented with beneficial microorganisms or probiotics—raw materials made up of high amounts of beneficial bioactive alkaloids.

I know this is a lot of technical information, and Grandma Rose didn't understand everything I was explaining either. After reviewing my list and taking a long swallow, however, she approved the direction I was taking her in. Then again, she knew she had knocked on death's door, so she was vitally interested in giving her body the best chance possible to fight off this deadly disease.

I reminded Grandma Rose that my research on vitamins A, C, E, and beta-carotene showed that vitamin C protected the body from the damaging effects of toxins; vitamin E was effective against bowel and breast cancer; and vitamin A and beta-carotene were powerful antioxidants that prevented the formation of ions that damage the cells' DNA, which is one way that cancer spreads.

The transformation in Grandma Rose's health was dramatic after she started my nutritional supplement program. Not only did she gain weight, but she told everyone she met that her energy level, physical appearance, and general health were the best in thirty years. Within six months, a CAT scan revealed that she was cancer-free.

STEERING IN YOUR DIRECTION

I urge you to consider using nutritional supplements to fight cancer. Topping my list is a multivitamin fermented with probiotics known as *whole food* or *living* multivitamins. These vitamins contain different compounds such as organic acids, antioxidants, and key nutrients. They are more costly to produce since the ingredients—fruits, vegetables, vitamins, minerals, and so on—are put through a fermentation process similar to the digestive process of the body.

In addition to a whole food or living multivitamin, you should incorporate the following supplements into your daily nutrition plan.

High Omega-3 Cod-Liver Oil

A fishy-smelling liquid that people like to make fun of, cod-liver oil deserves greater respect because this superstar supplement delivers four nutrients that we hardly get enough of: eicosapentaenoic acid (EPA) and docosahexaenoic acid (DHA), vitamin A, and vitamin D.

EPA and DHA are long-chain polyunsaturated fats known as omega-3 fatty acids, and they are wonderful for your immune system. Dr. Johanna Budwig, nominated for the Nobel Prize numerous times, postulated that many diseases can proliferate because of insufficient good fats in the diet. With regard to cancer, omega-3 fats allow the body to utilize oxygen more efficiently, which is important because cancer cannot exist in the presence of oxygen. If you can use more oxygen by taking in omega-3 fats, your energy will increase, and your immune system will be better equipped to fight disease more effectively. A study in the *Journal of Nutrition* concluded that "consumption of omega-3 fatty acids might slow or stop the growth of metastatic cancer cells, increase longevity of cancer patients, and improve their quality of life."[1]

Cod-liver oil also contains more vitamin A per unit weight than other common foods, and its high levels of vitamin D are helpful in preventing cancer. Don't let the fishy taste keep you from introducing this nutrient into your diet. These days, cod-liver oil comes in lemon mint and other flavors that mask the odor and taste.

Enzymes

Many early proponents of natural health—Bernard Jensen, Ph.D., Edward Howell, M.D., and William Kelley, D.D.S.—recommended the consumption of large amounts of digestive enzymes to aid in the digestion of food *and* free up the body's metabolic and lytic enzymes to break down any foreign material in the body. In this case, that would be cancer cells. Upon my grandmother's diagnosis of cancer, she went on a seven-day raw juice fast supplemented with large amounts of plant-based digestive enzymes.

Green Foods

Common vegetables like garlic, onions, broccoli, cabbage, and sprouts are some of the top healing foods for cancer, yet another form ranks right up there: green food concentrates, also known as green superfoods.

These superfoods are supercharged concentrates of vegetables such as spinach, kale, and parsley, in addition to the microalgaes like chlorella and spirulina, and sea vegetables like kelp. Superfoods, mixed in water or juice or sold as green drinks, are considered nutraceuticals because they allow the body to heal itself. Superfoods are close cousins to dark green leafy vegetables, and they offer great nutrient density and beneficial phytonutrients, which aid the body's immune response.

If you mix a couple of scoops of dried green food powder into a glass of water or juice (or swallow a handful of green superfood caplets), you will be drinking one of the most nutrient-dense foods on this green earth. One of the main ingredients, spirulina, contains beta-carotene and the blue pigment phycocyanin, which is a well-studied immune enhancer.

Whole Food Fiber Blend with Flaxseeds

A whole food fiber blend supplies your body with a nutrient-dense source of dietary fiber. Dietary fiber is a source of carbohydrates that can't be digested. The link between a high-fiber diet and colon cancer is the subject of debate in the medical community, but common sense tells me that moving toxic material, for lack of a better word, through the bowels faster is good for the body. If there is an overabundance of toxins in your digestive tract, a whole food fiber blend with flaxseeds can keep things moving along.

Green Tea

Here's another "green" food that has cancer-fighting substances called polyphenols, which appear to slow down the growth of prostate cancer cells.[2] (Black tea has similar properties.) Rochester University researchers discovered that chemicals in green tea shut down a key molecule, known as the aryl hydrocarbon (AH), which can play a significant role in the development of cancer.[3]

Protein Powder

Cancer patients often don't feel like eating, but they will sip a smoothie for sustenance. Although mixing protein powder into a fruit smoothie is a wonderful idea, you should be aware that commercially made protein powder usually is derived from soy, milk, or whey protein, and that's not so healthy for you. Most protein powders are highly processed and derived from cows injected with hormones and fed antibiotic grain or from genetically modified soybeans. You'll find many whey- or soy-based protein powders contain artificial sweeteners, flavorings, and additives.

The healthier option is choosing whey protein powders from grass-fed, free-range cows, fermented soy protein, or my favorite—a protein powder made from goat's milk.

Probiotics

By definition, probiotics are living, direct-fed microbials, or DFMs, that promote the growth of beneficial bacteria in the intestinal tract. What happens is that the probiotics crowd out disease-causing bacteria, viruses, and yeasts, thus freeing the immune system to battle the cancer cells instead of the germs.

Resveratrol

This antioxidant, found in grapes and red wines, has been found to protect the skin cells from damages that may lead to the development of cancer.[4]

Herbs and Spices

The judicious use of the correct herbs can support the immune system and prevent cancer. The National Library of Medicine's database points out that ginger, turmeric, green or black tea, and flaxseed contain potent phytochemicals, which provide significant protection against cancer.[5] Garlic interferes with the ability of cancer-causing chemicals to damage DNA. Mint contains limonene, a powerful anticancer agent.

I mentioned the importance of foods high in beta-carotene. Basil, coriander, dill, fennel leaves, mint, parsley, and rosemary are among the herbs and spices highest in beta-carotene.

CHECK OUT SELENIUM

The mineral selenium is catching some attention for its cancer-fighting abilities. Several human studies suggest that selenium, an essential mineral found in most plant foods and nuts, may reduce the risk of lung, colorectal, gastrointestinal, and bladder cancer, but at least one study suggests it may prevent cancer more effectively in men than in women. We'll know more of selenium's effectiveness with prostate cancer when the results of a major National Cancer Institute study are released in several years.[6]

Modern medicine is looking to nature's bounty in the search for cancer cures. The National Cancer Institute has collected approximately 100,000 plant and marine samples from around the world. The samples are crushed into powder and made into extracts that are tested against human cancer cells. "The complexity and diversity of natural products can't be matched by even the most innovative human scientist," said Greg Vite of Bristol-Myers Squibb. "I think we're going to see a resurgence of interest in natural products."[7]

So do I.

Nutrient Depletions in Conventional Cancer Therapies

If you're among those taking one of the more than one thousand different chemotherapeutic agents or enduring invasive radiation, be aware that these treatments deplete the body of important nutrients. Frederic Vagnani, M.D., and Barry Fox, Ph.D., authors of *The Side Effects Bible*, compiled a list of these depleted nutrients and the dosage ranges you should consider taking in whole food vitamin and mineral supplement form.[8] I have modified the list by allowing for the supplementation of whole food nutrients, which are more bioavailable and thus can be consumed in smaller amounts.

- calcium: 600 mg/day suggested
- magnesium: 250–500 mg/day suggested
- potassium: 99 mg/day suggested
- riboflavin: 25 mg/day suggested
- coenzyme Q-10: 30 mg/day suggested
- thiamine: 25 mg/day suggested
- vitamin B_6: 25 mg/day suggested
- vitamin B_{12}: 500 mcg/day suggested
- beta-carotene: 5,000–10,000 IU/day suggested (estimated recommendation based on new calculation for recommended daily allowance)

THE GREAT PHYSICIAN'S Rx FOR CANCER: SUPPLEMENT YOUR DIET WITH WHOLE FOOD NUTRITIONALS, LIVING NUTRIENTS, AND SUPERFOODS

- *Don't believe physicians who say that taking vitamins and minerals is a worthless effort in the fight against cancer.*

- *Consume a whole food multivitamin high in antioxidants each day.*

- *Take one-to-three teaspoons or three-to-nine capsules of high omega-3 cod-liver oil per day with dinner.*

- *Each morning and evening, drink a serving or take five caplets of a green superfood supplement and a whole food fiber blend that contains flaxseed.*

- *Consume high amounts of a plant-based digestive enzyme blend.*

- *Take probiotics to improve digestion and immune system health.*

- *To ensure optimal protein intake, incorporate an easily digestible protein powder into your daily diet.*

Take Action

To learn how to incorporate the principles of supplementing your diet with whole food nutritionals, living nutrients, and superfoods into your daily regimen, please turn to page 73 for the Great Physician's Rx for Cancer Battle Plan.

KEY #3

Practice Advanced Hygiene

Not long after my wife, Nicki, and I learned that we would become proud parents of a baby boy—thanks to an ultrasound in her fifth month—we put that information to good use. We finished decorating his bedroom in accents of baby blue, informed the family so they could buy the right clothes for the baby, and purchased his first baseball glove.

Okay, scratch that last item, but when I heard that we would be bringing a son into this world, I mentally prepared myself for Joshua's circumcision. The decision of whether to circumcise Joshua was a no-brainer for two reasons:

1. In Genesis 17:10–14, God directed Abraham to circumcise himself, his household, and his slaves as part of an everlasting covenant in which God promised to make Abraham the father of a multitude of nations.

2. I believe God's Word is always backed up by science, and if the Creator ordained circumcision on the eighth day of a boy's life, then I know He had His reasons.

We had Joshua circumcised in our home by a *mohel* (pronounced *moyle*), usually a Jewish rabbi or physician who performs the religious ceremony/medical procedure. The cutting away of his tiny foreskin wasn't easy to watch, but I felt great satisfaction knowing that I was fulfilling a directive from God and welcoming Joshua into a family that included Abraham, Isaac, Jacob, Moses,

Joshua, David, and our Savior Jesus, as well as my male ancestors. Both of my parents are Jewish, but when I was born, Dad was in naturopathic school, where he was taught that circumcision was a barbaric practice unnecessary in today's enlightened times. Fortunately, someone convinced him I should be circumcised, and that happened when I was around three weeks old.

From what I hear, though, circumcision—whether performed as part of a *bris milah* ceremony or in a doctor's office—is on the wane these days. Over the past twenty years, the rates of hospital circumcision have fallen steadily as parents wonder whether they should allow their son's foreskin—the sensitive sleeve of skin covering the head of the penis—to be snipped away.

Twenty-five years ago, researchers believe that as many as 85 percent of baby boys in the United States were circumcised. By 2003 that figure had dropped to 56 percent, and according to the National Center for Health Statistics, less than 37 percent of boys born in hospitals in western states were circumcised.[1] A noisy group of circumcision protesters have picketed hospitals in recent years, carrying signs that read, "Peace begins with how we treat our children." Adult men claiming that they were sexually desensitized without their consent or that their parents were not fully informed before signing consent papers have filed lawsuits.

I'm afraid these well-meaning folks are misguided. As I said, God knew what He was doing when He introduced circumcision to His chosen people, although I would imagine that the idea of slicing off a part of your manhood sounded pretty far out to Abraham, who was ninety-nine years old at the time. God required circumcision as a sign of obedience and as a visible sign that identified the male as a child of God forever. There was no way to reverse this procedure.

Some biblical scholars say that circumcision was a symbol of "cutting off" the old life of sin, but I believe God instituted the practice for health reasons as well; otherwise, why did He specifically say that newborn males must be circumcised on the eighth day of life? Modern medicine has discovered that the eighth day is an ideal time for a circumcision. Vitamin K, a necessary component for blood clotting, is normally at low levels in newborns, but this clotting agent rises *above* adult levels around the seventh day of life before settling in at adult levels around day ten. God had specific reasons for designating Day 8 as the best time to circumcise male newborns.

What also interests me is that modern medicine has established a link between circumcision and cancer. For instance, the overall rate of penile cancer in this country is low—about one case per 100,000 men—but when researchers studied eighty-nine men with invasive penile cancer, eighty-seven men, or 97 percent, had not been circumcised.[2]

In addition, women are less likely to develop cancer of the cervix if they are in a sexual relationship with a circumcised male rather than an uncircumcised male.[3] Circumcised men were half as likely to be infected with HPV, or human papillomavirus, a sexually transmitted disease.[4] HPV can cause cervical cancer.

If you're an uncircumcised male, I'm not suggesting that you look up *mohels* in the yellow pages and schedule a *bris* posthaste, but you should be aware that being uncircumcised puts you, as well as your spouse, at greater risk for certain types of cancers.

INTRODUCING ADVANCED HYGIENE

Your body will be better prepared to fight off cancer if you practice advanced hygiene, which will protect you from germs that challenge the body's immune system. Many of us forget that bacteria, viruses, fungi, and other germs mount attacks on the body's cellular network around the clock. The immune system repels these assaults with battalions of microscopic foot soldiers: T cells, B cells, macrophages, and eosinophils. If these defensive forces are overwhelmed, however, the body is vulnerable to various illnesses. In such a scenario, dangerous cancer cells could gain a beachhead.

Proper hygiene supports your immune system in this constant battle against germs and foreign agents entering the body. That's why I've included it as one of the seven keys in *The Great Physician's Rx for Cancer*. In some ways, proper advanced hygiene can be just as important as diet and exercise in the pursuit of good health.

Hygiene literally means "conditions and practices that serve to promote or preserve health." By regularly practicing advanced hygiene, you can significantly reduce infections, allergy attacks, and other negative health conditions by cleansing your body of toxins, pollutants, disease-causing germs, and allergens.

I've been practicing an advanced hygiene protocol for more than a decade and have been the beneficiary of excellent health: no lingering head colds, no nagging sinus infections, and no acute respiratory illnesses to speak of for many years. I'm also confident that advanced hygiene is a superior *long-term weapon* against cancer ever gaining a foothold within my body.

I follow a program first developed by an Australian scientist,

Kenneth Seaton, Ph.D., who discovered that ear, nose, throat, and skin problems could be linked to the fact that humans touch the nose, eyes, and mouth with germ-carrying fingernails throughout the day. If you thought that most germs were spread by airborne exposure—someone sneezing at your table—you would be wrong. "Germs don't fly; they hitchhike," Dr. Seaton declared, and I believe he's right.

We pick up germs through everyday actions: shaking hands with others or touching handrails, doorknobs, shopping carts, paper money, coins, and food. One can become rather paranoid thinking of all the possibilities of routine contact with germs, and I choose not to go that route. I prefer to go through life without washing my hands until they're red raw in a compulsive fashion.

At the same time, however, I'm aware that 90 percent of germs on my hands take up residence underneath my fingernails, so I use a creamy semisoft soap rich in essential oils each morning and evening. To properly wash my hands, I dip them into the tub of semisoft soap and dig my fingernails into the cream. Then I work the special cream around the tips of fingers, cuticles, and fingernails for fifteen to thirty seconds. When I'm finished, I lather my hands for fifteen seconds before rinsing them under running water. After my hands are clean, I take another dab of semisoft soap and wash my face.

My second step involves a procedure that I call a facial dip. I fill my washbasin or a clean, large bowl with warm but not hot water. When enough water is in the basin, I add a tablespoon or two of regular table salt and two eyedroppers of a mineral-based facial solution into the cloudy water. I mix everything up with my hands, and then I bend over and dip my face into the cleansing solution, opening my eyes several times to allow the membranes to be cleaned. After coming up for air, I dunk my head a second time and blow bubbles through my nose. "Sink snorkeling," I call it.

My final two steps of advanced hygiene involve applying very diluted drops of hydrogen peroxide and minerals into my ears for thirty to sixty seconds to cleanse the ear canal and then brushing my teeth with an essential oil-based tooth solution to cleanse my mouth of unhealthy germs.

Albumin to the Rescue

Chances are that you've never heard of the most abundant protein in the bloodstream—albumin, which transports hormones, nutrients, and wastes throughout the body. Like a dump truck on its way to the landfill, albumin hauls wastes and toxic cells to the liver for degradation and elimination from the body. Because this protein sails through the bloodstream to every part of the body, cancer researchers have looked for ways to bind cancer-fighting particles to albumin. They've discovered how to perform this remarkable feat. The drug Abraxane, approved by the U.S. Food and Drug Administration in 2005 to fight breast cancer, was shown to successfully attach paclitaxel particles—or anticancer agents—to albumin.[5]

Medical researchers have also discovered another interesting bit of news: high albumin levels may be critical to the prevention of diseases like cancer. Cancer patients, when tested, have low albumin levels. How this relates to cancer is still being researched, but doctors believe that those with low albumin levels *before* cancer strikes could be at greater risk.

That's why Dr. Seaton is certain that albumin levels are linked to *hygiene,* not diet, meaning that albumin levels can be optimized by practicing advanced hygiene, which underscores the importance of this key as part of *The Great Physician's Rx for Cancer.*

You need to be aware that the first demonstrated cure for cancer was based on hygiene, and it dates back to the eighteenth century when Dr. Percival Potts, a British physician, discovered the connection between scrotal cancer and chimney sweeps, who worked in dreadfully dirty and smoky conditions. After the sweeps spent years of toiling in cramped, ash-encrusted quarters, Dr. Potts noticed that black soot collected in the folds of the scrotal skin—the same place where cancerous tumors formed. Because indoor plumbing was a rarity for the working class, chimney sweeps—like the rest of the English populace—bathed once a week, at best. Without proper hygiene, the carcinogenic properties of the soot dissolved into the skin and caused cancer to form.

When Danish doctors heard about Dr. Potts's pioneering work, they convinced Danish chimney sweeps to wear protective clothing *and* wash themselves more often than on Saturday nights. Scrotal cancer rates for Danish chimney sweeps plunged after the cancer-producing soot and ashes were washed away regularly. Meanwhile, British chimney sweeps continued to develop cancer in droves because they couldn't—or wouldn't—embrace improved hygienic habits.

That's why I urge you to embrace advanced hygiene with the understanding that battling everyday germs today can help you be cancer-free tomorrow.

℞ THE GREAT PHYSICIAN'S Rx FOR CANCER: PRACTICE ADVANCED HYGIENE

- *Wash your hands regularly, paying special attention to removing germs from underneath your fingernails.*

- *Cleanse your nasal passageways and the mucous membranes of the eyes daily by performing a facial dip.*

- *Cleanse the ear canals at least twice per week.*

- *Use an essential oil–based tooth solution daily to remove germs from the mouth.*

Take Action

To learn how to incorporate the principles of practicing advanced hygiene into your daily regimen, please turn to page 73 for the Great Physician's Rx for Cancer Battle Plan.

KEY #4

Condition Your Body
with Exercise and Body Therapies

Were you aware that the prestigious Stanford Cancer Institute, known worldwide for its sterling care and cutting-edge treatments for cancer, calls exercise an "alternative therapy" on its Web site? It's true; exercise is lumped together with biofeedback and hypnosis. "Scientists are still learning about how physical activity helps cancer patients and what impact it has on the immune system," declares the Web site.

Well, the Stanford Cancer Institute may want to update its advice because elsewhere, the medical community is wising up to the benefits of exercise in regard to cancer. *The Journal of the American Medical Association* (*JAMA*) reported in 2005 that walking just three to five hours a week could boost a woman's chance of surviving breast cancer by 50 percent.[1] Another study released in 2005 by the Dana-Farber Institute found a 40 to 50 percent reduction in the recurrence of stage III colon cancer for those who undertook an exercise program following chemotherapy.[2]

If you just learned you have cancer, I suggest you get going and get walking—and you don't have to break any speed records. In the aforementioned breast cancer study, women reported walking at an average pace—not like an Olympian race walker. The point is that slow but steady walking is an effective load-bearing exercise that places a gentle strain on the hips and the rest of the body. Doctors believe that exercises such as walking lower hormone levels, and lower hormonal levels reduce the chances of cancer recurring in the body. A Penn State study determined that women with breast cancer who participated in moderate aerobic activities such as walking or pedaling an exercise bike experienced an increase in infection-fighting T cells.[3]

The reason why I like walking so much is that this exercise can be performed anytime or anywhere, alone or with friends. The last thing you want to do when you have cancer is retreat to the couch with a down-and-out attitude. Call your friends and ask them to join you for a purposeful twilight walk. You need to do some sort of physical activity because if you don't, you'll experience a loss of movement and function. The old "use it or lose it" syndrome still applies.

Modest amounts of exertion can accomplish the following for cancer patients:

- reduce anxiety or depression
- reduce fatigue
- improve blood flow to the legs and reduce the risk of blood clots
- reduce pain
- reduce diarrhea or constipation
- prevent osteoporosis
- reduce the risk of heart disease
- increase overall physical functioning

- reduce dependence on others for the activities of daily living

- improve self-esteem[4]

I incorporate a form of personal exercise into my life that should be very beneficial to cancer patients as well as those aiming to *prevent* cancer. My preferred way to maintain a healthy body, increase strength, and improve flexibility is called *functional fitness,* which can be used as a therapy to restore the body to good health.

This form of gentle exercise can be performed within the privacy of your home and will get your body burning calories and improve agility. The idea behind functional fitness is to train movements, not muscles, as you exercise the cardiovascular system and the body's core muscles. You do this through performing real-life activities in real-life positions.

Functional fitness can be done with no equipment or with dumbbells, mini trampolines, and stability balls. You can find functional fitness classes and equipment at gyms around the country, including LA Fitness, Bally Total Fitness, and local YMCAs. You'll be asked to perform squats with feet apart, feet together, and one back with the other forward. You'll be asked to do reaching lunges, push-ups against a wall, and "supermans" that involve lying on the floor and lifting up your right arm while lifting your left leg into a fully extended position. You *won't* be asked to perform high-impact exercises like those found in pulsating aerobics classes.

I believe that a functional fitness program effectively combats the fatigue that cancer patients feel after undergoing chemotherapy and radiation treatment. Around 80 percent of chemotherapy patients said they experienced noticeable fatigue after their first and second cycles of treatment.[5] (For more information on functional fitness, visit www.GreatPhysiciansRx.com.)

YOU SHOULD SLEEP ON IT

Exercise is one of the many body therapies beneficial to cancer patients and those actively seeking to prevent cancer from striking. A good night's sleep, according to a Stanford University Medical Center study, may influence cancer progression. The brain churns out a hormone known as melatonin, which has antioxidant properties. The body's antioxidants have an important job: mopping up the dangerous free radicals lying in wait to wreak havoc on the body's tissues and organs. When you don't sleep enough, melatonin production is hindered, along with the hormone cortisol. The Stanford study cited the ability of melatonin and cortisol to regulate the activities of the immune system and the cells that fight off cancerous cells.[6]

How much sleep do you need? The goal should be eight hours, which would be around an hour more than what the average American adult receives these days, according to the National Sleep Foundation. Why the magic number of eight hours? Because when people are allowed to "sleep out" and wake up when they want to under controlled laboratory conditions, they generally sleep eight hours in a twenty-four-hour period. This

where the word *melanoma* has become a household word and worried moms slather their children with oily creams containing sun protection factors (SPFs) of 30, lest their sons and daughters develop a dangerous form of skin cancer. But think about it: Why are we experiencing higher rates of skin cancer today when we spend 90 percent of our time indoors (according to the research I've seen) and our ancestors—who toiled outside from sunup to sundown—didn't get skin cancer in nearly the same rates as today?

My answer is that we lack adequate nutrients in our diets and don't eat enough antioxidant-rich fruits, vegetables, and healthy fats, which naturally protect us from skin cancer. I urge you to incorporate sunbathing into your daily routine, *especially* if you are fighting cancer. The National Institutes of Health (NIH) state that all you need is ten to fifteen minutes of sunlight for vitamin D synthesis to occur.

I'm pleased that the mainstream media are seeing the light, so to speak, and are agreeing with me. "A Neglected Nutrient: Are Americans Dying from a Lack of Vitamin D?" asked a *Newsweek* article.[7] "Making a Case for Sun's Benefits," declared a *Los Angeles Times* headline. The latter story, which called vitamin D the "sunshine vitamin," pointed toward studies suggesting that vitamin D was responsible for reducing the risk of lymphoma, improving the survival rate of lung cancer, and contributing to the decline of skin cancer, which the writer found "ironic."[8]

Not me. I didn't raise an eyebrow when I heard that Dr. Edward Giovannucci, a Harvard University professor of medicine and nutrition, announced at a recent American Association for Cancer Research meeting that his research suggests that vitamin

D from sunlight might prevent thirty deaths for each one caused by the sun.[9]

A MAGNIFICENT QUARTET

Allow me to quickly introduce four other valuable body therapies.

1. Hydrotherapy

With a Latin root of *hydro,* this body therapy involves the use of water in various ways: baths, showers, ice, and steam. Types of hydrotherapy include whirlpool baths for relaxation, ice packs to reduce swelling, warm and cold water for cleansing, and steam baths to alleviate stress.

Heat-based therapies, such as sitting in hot water or saunas, cause the blood vessels to dilate, which boosts circulation and speeds the elimination of toxins. Cold-based therapies, on the other hand, constrict blood vessels, decrease swelling, and boost oxygen use in the cells. The simplest form of hot-cold hydrotherapy is one I regularly practice: taking a hot shower, followed by turning the water ice cold for up to a minute.

The healing properties of water can be a soothing balm to a body fighting cancer and an excellent way to increase energy at a time when you need a boost. The American Cancer Society calls hydrotherapy an effective complementary therapy.

2. Aromatherapy

Chances are that you haven't heard much about this body therapy involving the sense of smell and the use of essential oils in a variety of healing ways. Today, aromatherapy means the application of highly concentrated oils distilled from plants such as myrtle, coriander, hyssop, galbanum, and rosemary. These plants are among the 188 references to precious oils in Scripture, including James 5:14 (NLT), which states, "Are any among you sick? They should call for the elders of the church and have them pray over them, anointing them with oil in the name of the Lord."

I believe extensive health benefits can be derived from introducing essential oils to your skin and pores. You may drop an eyedropper of essential oils into hot bathwater, burn them in a diffuser, or rub a few drops on your fingers, cup your hands over your mouth and nose, and inhale a deep breath.

Aromatherapy may not slow the growth of cancer, but you'll feel better for having tried it. While there is no scientific proof, the American Cancer Society says that essential oils such as lemon fragrance and French basil could stimulate the immune system. *The Encyclopedia of Natural Healing* recommends bergamot oil, cypress oil, eucalyptus oil, geranium oil, and lavender oil.[10]

3. Music Therapy

By definition, music therapy is listening to specific music to promote relaxation and healing. I can't speak from personal experience, but if I was sitting in a recliner while cancer-fighting drugs were injected into my arm, I would find listening to uplifting praise and worship music on my headphones to be calming and healing. Artists such as Steven Curtis Chapman, Casting Crowns, and Jeremy Camp or Hillsong praise and worship songs would be the ones I would have in my CD player or iPod.

4. Bibliotherapy

I can see the head-scratching going on: *What is bibliotherapy?* In Kirkless, West Yorkshire (that's in Great Britain), doctors and librarians teamed up to launch a program that puts "therapeutic novels" in the hands of patients suffering from a variety of ailments, including cancer.

With all the great Christian fiction on the bookshelves these days, I think an inspirational read will help anyone suffering from cancer feel as if he isn't being Left Behind. Okay, a bad joke, but I still like the concept of bibliotherapy, which can be traced back to ancient Greece, where the words "Medicine for the Soul" were etched in the marble façade over the door to the library at Thebes.

R_x **THE GREAT PHYSICIAN'S Rx FOR CANCER: CONDITION YOUR BODY WITH EXERCISE AND BODY THERAPIES**

- *Make a commitment to exercise at least three times a week, either at a fitness center or by walking close to home or work.*

- *Incorporate five to fifteen minutes of functional fitness into your daily schedule.*

- *Go to sleep earlier, paying close attention to how much sleep you get before midnight. Do your best to get eight hours of sleep nightly. Remember that sleep* is the most important nonnutrient thing you can do for your health.

- End your next shower by changing the water temperature to cool (or cold) and standing underneath the spray for one minute.

- Take a magazine (or this book!), and during your next break from work, sit outside in a chair and face the sun. Soak up the rays for ten or fifteen minutes (but be careful between 10:00 a.m. and 2:00 p.m.).

- Play worship music in your home, in your car, or on your iPod. Now's the time to focus on what's really important.

Take Action

To learn how to incorporate the principles of conditioning your body with exercise and body therapies into your daily regimen, please turn to page 73 for the Great Physician's Rx for Cancer Battle Plan.

KEY #5

Reduce Toxins in Your Environment

If you were to do a word association game with someone, chances are high that after you uttered the word *toxins,* he would quickly respond with "cancer." In a post-Chernobyl planet, people intuitively understand the cancer risk associated with toxins in our environment. Many of us are aware that we live in a toxic world where the prudent should protect themselves from chemicals, pollutants, and industrial compounds present in the food we eat, the air we breathe, the water we drink, and the everyday household products we come into physical contact with.

The problem is that it's impossible *not* to come into close contact with potential carcinogens in our environment, unless we want to go through life like John Travolta did in the 1970s tearjerker movie *The Boy in the Plastic Bubble.* The following is a list of what the National Toxicology Program and Environmental Protection Agency have labeled as cancer-causing agents:

- PCBs, or polychlorinated biphenyls, are found in paint, ink, and dye, but more important, PCB concentrations also reside in the fatty tissues of land animals and fish. For instance, farm-raised salmon, popular in supermarkets, warehouse clubs, and restaurants, are raised on pellets of ground-up fish that absorb PCBs from the environment.

55

- Dioxins are harmful compounds used in the manufacturing of plastic and PVC piping. There's a worry that plastic containers may release dioxins when superheated in microwave ovens. While there is no strong evidence implicating plastic containers as a threat to humans, I wouldn't microwave leftovers in plastic containers, which are made from petroleum-based compounds. If you must use the microwave oven (I don't have one, and I recommend that anyone with cancer completely avoid them), then put your food on a microwave-safe plate and cover it with paper towels or waxed paper. Whatever you do, don't use plastic wrap (which may contain dioxins) or let it come in contact with your food.

- Trace particles of arsenic can be found in tap water.[1]

I suggest that you drink as much bottled or filtered water as possible. Not all bottled waters are created equally, however. Some brands are nothing more than purified tap water, which means they may not be much safer or healthier than water straight from the tap. I would shop for spring waters such as Arrowhead, Deer Park, or Poland Spring; they are drawn from underground sources and thus considered more pristine.

Nearly all municipal water is treated with chlorine, a substance that may be carcinogenic and is certainly toxic because of its disinfectant ability to kill bacteria and algae. Installing a water filtration system in your home means you'll receive filtered water every time you turn on the tap, but these systems run several thousand dollars. A more modest investment of twenty dollars for a countertop water pitcher with a carbon-based filter will suffice.

Did you know that when you take a steaming hot shower, your skin absorbs the equivalent of six to eight glasses of chlorinated water? A shower filter will protect your body from absorbing the chlorine. That's why I strongly urge the installation of shower filters with kinetic degradation fluxion (KDF) units that remove chlorine, heavy metals, and bacteria from the water.

When you're not under a shower, drink lots of water . . . *lots* of water. Doing this will give your body the physiological ability to flush out toxins from its system. God, in His infinite wisdom, designed the body to quickly get rid of water-soluble chemical toxins, but fat-soluble chemicals such as dioxins are stored in our fatty tissues and can take months or years before they're successfully eliminated from our systems. Flushing your body with copious amounts of water will rid you of those toxins earlier.

Fat-soluble toxins are created by the chemical residues residing inside your body, which scientists refer to as a person's *total body burden*. How much body burden is too much? What's the tipping point when your body burden is so great that you can no longer destroy cancer cells?

Nobody's sure, and that's a problem because in a study led by Mount Sinai School of Medicine in New York, in collaboration with the Environmental Working Group and Commonwealth, researchers at two major laboratories found an average of ninety-one industrial compounds, pollutants, and other chemicals in the blood and urine of nine volunteers.[2]

SOME STRATEGIES

If you have received a cancer diagnosis, let me state something boldly and directly: you need to eat natural and preferably organic foods. This is not an option. Commercially grown fruits and vegetables are routinely sprayed with herbicides and pesticides while organic foodstuffs, by definition, are grown without the use of toxic pesticides and fertilizers. Don't take any chances; no matter where you purchase your fruits and veggies—a supermarket, health food store, or farmer's roadside stand—you should thoroughly wash your food just to be safe.

Organic foods are much more than sweet melons, leafy green lettuce, or plump red tomatoes fresh from the vine. When I talk about organic foods, I'm referring to cereals, dairy products, and meats coming from livestock that graze on unsprayed fields of grass and are fed with organic feed. Yes, it will cost more to shop at places like Whole Foods, Wild Oats, or your local natural health food store, but this is not the time to be pinching dollars.

Besides drinking natural spring water and installing carbon filters at your kitchen sink and shower outlets, you should take steps to purify the air in your living space. Today's well-insulated homes and energy-efficient windows and doors trap "used" air with harmful particles of carbon dioxide, nitrogen dioxide, and pet dander. When the U.S. Environmental Protection Agency (EPA) conducted a survey of six hundred homes in six cities, researchers discovered that peak concentrations of twenty toxic compounds were hundreds of times higher *inside* homes than outside. "If we measured outdoors what we are measuring indoors," said EPA spokesperson Lance Wallace, "there would be a tremendous cry to clean up outdoor air."[3]

Open your doors and windows to let fresh air flow into your home several times a day, no matter what the temperature is like outside. Even in Florida's sticky summer heat, Nicki and I periodically air out the house, and we sleep with a window cracked open in the master bedroom. We've also set up four air purifiers inside our home, which clean room air through electrical charges to capture airborne particles, microbes, and molds. Air purifiers are a wonderful technology that's becoming more affordable each year.

Indoor houseplants also absorb toxic compounds and pollutants. The National Aeronautics and Space Administration (NASA) performed a study showing that indoor plants such as English ivy, Chinese evergreen, and weeping fig can remove up to 87 percent of the toxins contained in indoor air. Healthy, mature indoor plants not only clean up your indoor environment, but they add a lovely green accent to home furnishings.

In some parts of the country, a radon test is part of a home inspection before someone buys a home. Radon is a colorless, odorless gas that can be carcinogenic, and when radon levels are higher than U.S. government standards, the house sellers are usually asked to pay for additional venting into the home—further proof that fresh air is a welcome antidote to toxins in the air we breathe.

AROUND THE HOUSE

Carcinogenic contaminants are found in a variety of popular household products, including cleaners and cosmetics. Regarding the former, the less contact with kitchen cleansers, oven cleaners, glues, paints, paint thinners, and other solvents, the better.

Regarding the latter, cosmetics, hair dyes, and hair sprays have toxic qualities. Natural cosmetics can be found in progressive groceries and natural food stores nationwide, or visit www.BiblicalHealthInstitute.com and click on the GPRx Resource Guide.

Let me leave you with this thought regarding toxins in your environment: as a defense, some scientists will quote Paracelsus, the famous medieval alchemist, who said hundreds of years ago, "It's the dose that makes the poison." In other words, if the toxic dose is low enough, the body can handle it.

When I look at today's cancer statistics, it's apparent that we are being hit with too many toxic doses from too many areas in our environment, and that's why we must be proactive in reducing toxins in our personal environments.

R̶x̶ THE GREAT PHYSICIAN'S Rx FOR CANCER: REDUCE TOXINS IN YOUR ENVIRONMENT

- *Consume organically produced food as much as possible.*

- *Improve indoor air quality by opening windows, changing air filters regularly, setting out house-plants, and buying an air filtration system.*

- *Drink only purified water.*

- *Shower in purified water.*

- *Use natural products for skin care, body care, hair care, and cosmetics.*

- *Don't heat food in plastic.*

- *Don't cook with microwave ovens.*

- *Use natural cleaning products for your home, washing machine, and dishwasher.*

- *Don't smoke cigarettes or use tobacco products.*

Take Action

To learn how to incorporate the principles of reducing toxins in your environment into your daily regimen, please turn to page 73 for the Great Physician's Rx for Cancer Battle Plan.

KEY #6

Avoid Deadly Emotions

They say that a person can live thirty days without food, three days without water, three minutes without air, and thirty seconds without hope.

That may be an exaggeration, but I do know that you can't live long without hope, and I don't know how those who *don't* have the hope that comes from the Lord manage to get through a single day. I once heard about an underground U.S. government study in which medical physicians informed a group of *healthy* people—and this will sound horrible—that they had six months to live. Half of the study group were dead six months later.

This may sound like Area 51 stuff, but whether true or not, I'm aware of the roller-coaster emotions that one experiences when an oncologist says to "put your affairs in order." You see, I was near death about ten years ago when my body was losing a huge struggle with various life-threatening diseases. At twenty years of age, my extremely fit body had wasted away to 104 pounds, and I looked like a death camp refugee. I overheard a crying nurse tell another nurse, "This young man isn't going to make it through the night."

I closed my eyes and, with a resigned heart, spoke with God. "Lord," I began, "I'm ready to go home. I don't want to be in this body if life is going to be like this." I fell asleep, not knowing if I would wake up in the morning, but I did. Even though

I rallied, I was ready for anything that would come. I'll never forget boarding an airplane on the way to another clinic and looking out the window as the ground crew finished loading the bags. *If this plane went down, it wouldn't be too bad,* I thought.

I had reached the point of acceptance, the last of the classic "five stages of grief" as articulated by Elisabeth Kübler-Ross in her seminal book, *On Death and Dying* (Scribner, 1997). The five stages are these:

1. denial
2. anger
3. bargaining
4. depression
5. acceptance

After denying my condition for months, I can remember the sheer anger I felt at God for allowing me to become deathly ill. Why would He do that to me? I had believed in Jesus for my salvation at a young age and had served Him faithfully in my teen years and right into my freshman year of college at Florida State University, where I was majoring in preministerial communications. Just before my sophomore year, however, I was struck by around-the-clock diarrhea, horrible cramps, and knifelike thrusts into my abdomen.

As my health rapidly deteriorated, I directed seething anger at God, but that didn't last long because I became eager to bargain with my Creator—that's how desperate I was to be healed.

In fact, I told God that if He healed me, I would make it my life's mission to share what I learned about health with the world.

But as months dragged into years, I dealt with the throes of deep depression, the fourth stage. When I became resigned to my fate—a marginal life wearing colostomy bags or an early death—I accepted whatever the Lord, the Author of life, had in store for my life and, yes, even death.

If you are in the midst of health challenges or have received such a disheartening diagnosis, my heart goes out to you. Words escape me, and perhaps your family members don't know what to say either. It's beyond the scope of this book to delve deeper into the emotional pain that you may be enduring; for that, I urge you to speak with a counselor, your pastor, and trusted and loyal friends. What I hope to remind you about in this chapter is how deadly emotions can quickly deplete your dwindling reserves of energy and strength, especially if you are still dealing with depression and anger issues.

The connection between emotions and cancer cannot be overstated. Since cancer thrives upon a depressed immune system, your emotional attitude can affect the outcome of the disease. An entire journal, the *Psycho-Oncology Journal,* is dedicated to the study of emotions and cancer, but a better resource would be the Bible. Proverbs 14:30 tells us that envy brings rottenness to the bones, while Proverbs 17:22 states, "A merry heart does good, like medicine, but a broken spirit dries the bones."

Of course it's important to keep up your spirits, but what do bones have to do with cancer? The stem cells of some of your most important immune cells (the B and T cells) originate in the bone marrow. Steven Locke, M.D., of Harvard University completed a study that demonstrated how natural killer cell activity (responsible for destroying abnormal cells) decreased when patients exhibited symptoms of high stress in their lives.[1]

This finding doesn't surprise me. Don Colbert, M.D. and author of *Deadly Emotions,* states that the mind and body are closely linked, and the way you feel emotionally can determine how you feel physically. Certain emotions release hormones that can exacerbate your poor health—or help you recover.

Dr. Colbert believes, as I do, that a late-stage cancer diagnosis causes people to focus on what's truly important in their lives—God, their family, and other aspects of life that bring them deep peace and happiness. Perhaps you've experienced such clarity; if so, a terminal diagnosis has a way of clearing the emotional deck.

Since negative emotions release hormones that can trigger *more* cancer cell production, you should check your mental frame of mind. Are you harboring resentment at God because cancer is part of your life? Do you feel anger because your doctor didn't catch the disease earlier? Are you depressed when you consider the future?

These are deadly emotions that I urge you to confront, and feel free to invite a professional counselor to lead your introspection. While feelings of rage and resentment are expected, you need to address any lingering thoughts of unforgiveness in your heart.

I received a lesson about the importance of forgiving those who had hurt me from Dr. Bruce Wilkinson, author of the *Prayer of Jabez.* One morning, while we were sharing a breakfast meeting together, he dropped a thunderbolt out of the sky. "Jordan, is there anyone in your life that you need to forgive?" he inquired.

"I can't think of anyone," I replied, perhaps too quickly. Dr. Wilkinson knew I was giving him the polite brush-off, so he repeated his question about whether there was anyone in my life that I needed to forgive. As I contemplated his inquiry for a long moment, I thought back to those doctors who crushed my spirit when they said I had brought the illness upon myself in some way. Further reflection brought to mind several college friends who promised to call or write after I had to medically withdraw from college, but they disappeared from my life.

Dr. Wilkinson suggested that I write the names of the offending persons (although sometimes it's God or yourself you need to forgive) at the top of a piece of paper, followed by every grievance they brought against me. Then Dr. Wilkinson directed me to say, "I forgive [insert name] for doing [insert act]," just as God forgave me of my sins when Jesus willingly went to the cross for me. I did as he suggested, and after praying with a contrite heart, I ripped up the piece of paper and tossed it into the trash.

When you're dealing with cancer, or if a loved one is facing this life-threatening disease, I urge you to make amends and forgive those who have hurt you or caused you pain in the past. There's a reason why Paul wrote, "Don't let the sun go down while you are still angry" (Eph. 4:26 NLT). Feelings of fury and irritation are like an unquenchable fire that consumes everything in its path, causing bitterness and acrimony in its wake.

I witnessed for myself how a person's unwillingness to forgive can hasten death. For Grandma Rose, unforgiveness turned to bitterness in the last few years of life. She never forgave herself for mistreating my mother as a child due to her own miserable life. She never forgave God for the tough life she endured or for her sisters who died in the Holocaust. She had married young, and her husband had a hard time finding a job, so young Rose had to work like a horse performing menial jobs to keep the family going. Then her dying mother moved in with her. After that, a sister died, leaving behind two children, and those children moved in with Rose and her husband. Finally, I'm sure she also resented the fact that her husband died of a heart attack at the young age of fifty-five, leaving her a poor widow for nearly thirty years, forced to live off a modest Social Security check.

When Grandma Rose came down with cancer a second time, I rushed to Atlanta, where I asked her to write down the names of people she needed to forgive. She wouldn't do it. She thought it was more important that she ate healthy foods and took supplements than dealing with the people she needed to forgive. In the last six months of her life, I could see unforgiveness written all over the face of the grandmother I loved. If only she could have let go. If only she could have let God.

What about you? Is this the day you should take out a pad of paper and deal with the people you need to forgive? I hope so because the names you write down—and forgive in your heart of hearts—may give you many more years of life with those you love the most.

℞ THE GREAT PHYSICIAN'S Rx FOR CANCER: AVOID DEADLY EMOTIONS

- *Simplify your life and do your best to avoid stress, anxiety, and anger.*

- *Trust God when you face circumstances that cause you to worry or become anxious.*

- *Practice forgiveness every day and forgive those who have hurt you.*

- *Look for ways to laugh; it's your best medicine (Prov. 17:22).*

Take Action

To learn how to incorporate the principles of avoiding deadly emotions into your daily regimen, please turn to page 73 for the Great Physician's Rx for Cancer Battle Plan.

KEY #7

Live a Life of Prayer and Purpose

The phone call from my sister, Jenna, carried a sense of urgency. "Grandma is slipping away. If you want to see her again . . . ," she said, her voice trailing off.

I had to work hard to deal with my schedule—canceling business trips, rearranging meetings—but I knew I had to fly to Atlanta for the last few days of Grandma Rose's life.

My last visit was so poignant. Nicki and I brought along our son, Joshua, but I had heard that Grandma Rose had complained about the noise her other great-grandchild made on his visit, so we were genuinely concerned that seven-month-old Joshua would fuss and squirm and be asked to leave. Instead, he behaved very well, and Grandma Rose even sat up in her bed and rocked him in her pencil-thin arms.

"Look at this," she said and smiled. "He is so happy, and he's not even scared of the way I look." After a few moments, though, Grandma said to me, "Please take him away. I'm teasing him, and he's teasing me," as she handed our boy back to Nicki. A feeling of sadness came over me: my grandmother didn't have the energy to hug her infant great-grandson for more than a few minutes.

There was another reason why I cleared out my schedule to be there for Grandma Rose. Although my grandmother was born Jewish, she called herself an agnostic because she couldn't believe that God could allow such unspeakable horrors to be visited on her people by the Nazis. She didn't understand how a loving God could allow so much suffering in the world. Despite her misgivings, it was my profound hope that as she stood at the precipice of eternity, she would place her trust in Yeshua Ha Mashiach, the Messiah of the Jews, as her Savior.

"Grandma, can I sing you a song?" I asked during one visit. She weakly nodded for me to proceed, so I sang "Who Am I?" by Casting Crowns. It's one of my favorites, expressing wonder at how the Lord of all the earth knows our names and cares for each of us because we belong to Him. "Who am I? That the Lord of all the earth would care to know my name . . ."

The lyrics seemed appropriate to the moment, and that was my way of witnessing to her. I also read her comforting passages of Scripture.

I would love to write a happy ending . . . that Grandma Rose begged me to lead her through the "Sinner's Prayer" or that she raised her arms and cried out for the Lord. That didn't happen. And though she did not profess Jesus as Messiah before she left us, we believe there was a chance that God revealed Himself to her in the last two days when she couldn't speak, but only groaned. I made her promise that as she closed her eyes, she would run into the open arms of the Savior.

Grandma Rose has been gone for more than a year, but she has not been forgotten. Sharing her story gives me a renewed sense of purpose to help people suffering from cancer—or prevent this deadly disease from overtaking the body.

Cancer is a modern-day scourge, a lethal, scary disease in

our country. It's a horrible affliction that causes you to confront your mortality, and prayer is the most powerful tool we possess in the final fight against cancer. Prayer acknowledges that there is something . . . Someone . . . beyond the mortal confines of our lives. Talking to our Maker through prayer shouldn't be the treatment of last resort but the treatment of *first* resort. God may not answer our prayers in the way we expect Him to, but prayer will transform our hearts into greater alignment with His.

"Prayer must be foundational to every Christian endeavor," wrote Germaine Copeland, author of *Prayers That Avail Much*. Her book contains more than 150 prayers covering just about every situation under the sun: to receive Jesus as Lord and Savior (our prayer for Grandma Rose), healing for damaged emotions, victory over depression, and victory over fear. I was particularly drawn to Mrs. Copeland's prayer for "letting go of the past," since it resonated with Grandma Rose's situation:

Lord, I unfold my past and put into proper perspective those things that are behind. I trust in You, Lord, with all of my heart and lean not on my own understanding. Regardless of my past, I look forward to what lies ahead. I strain to reach the end of the race and receive the prize for which You are calling me up to heaven because of what Christ Jesus did for me. In His name I pray, amen.[1]

If you feel drawn to God at a crucial time like this, I urge you to get on your knees today. Prayer is imperative! Do not underestimate the power of communicating with your heavenly Father. When you pray and open up to God, you allow Him to fill your heart with Scripture, where He can speak to you in the stillness of the moment and transform your health simultaneously.

R THE GREAT PHYSICIAN'S Rx FOR CANCER: LIVE A LIFE OF PRAYER AND PURPOSE

- *Pray continually.*

- *Confess God's promises upon waking and before you retire.*

- *No matter where you are on your cancer journey, find God's purpose for your life and live it.*

Take Action

To learn how to incorporate the principles of living a life of prayer and purpose into your daily regimen, please turn to page 73 for the Great Physician's Rx for Cancer Battle Plan.

The Great Physician's Rx
for Cancer Battle Plan

Upon Waking and During the Daylight Hours

Prayer: thank God because this is the day that the Lord has made. Rejoice and be glad in it. Thank Him for the breath in your lungs and the life in your body. Ask the Lord to heal your body and use your experience to benefit the lives of others. Read Matthew 6:9–13 out loud.

Purpose: ask the Lord to give you an opportunity to add significance to someone's life today. Watch for that opportunity. Ask God to use you this day for His intended purpose.

Advanced hygiene: for hands and nails, jab fingers into semisoft soap four or five times, and lather hands with soap for fifteen seconds, rubbing soap over cuticles and rinsing under water as warm as you can stand. Take another swab of semisoft soap into your hands and wash your face. Next, fill the basin or sink with water as warm as you can stand it, and add one-to-three tablespoons of table salt and one-to-three eyedroppers of iodine-based mineral solution. Dunk face into water and open eyes, blinking repeatedly underwater. Keep eyes open underwater for three seconds. After cleaning your eyes, put your face back in the water, and close your mouth while blowing bubbles out of your nose. Come up from the water, and immerse your face in the water once again, gently taking water into your nostrils and expelling bubbles. Come up from the water, and blow your nose into facial tissue. To cleanse the ears, use hydrogen peroxide and mineral-based ear drops, putting two or three drops into each ear and letting stand for sixty seconds. Tilt your head to expel the drops. For the teeth, apply two or three drops of essential oil–based tooth drops to the toothbrush. This can be used to brush your teeth or added to existing toothpaste. After brushing your teeth, brush your tongue for fifteen seconds. (Visit www.BiblicalHealthInstitute.com and click on the GPRx Resource Guide for recommended advanced hygiene products.)

Reduce toxins: open your windows for one hour today. Use natural soap and natural skin and body care products (shower gel, body creams, etc.). Use natural facial care products. Use natural toothpaste. Use natural hair care products such as shampoo, conditioner, gel, mousse, and hairspray (visit www.BiblicalHealthInstitute.com and click on the GPRx Resource Guide for recommended hygiene products).

Body therapy: get twenty minutes of direct sunlight sometime during the day, but be careful between the hours of 10:00 a.m. and 2:00 p.m.

Exercise: try to walk outside in the fresh air, weather permitting, and finish with five or ten minutes of deep-breathing exercises (if you feel well enough to exercise).

Emotional health: whenever you face a circumstance, such as your health, that causes you to worry, repeat the following: "Lord, I trust You. I cast my cares upon You, and I believe that You're going to take care of [insert your current situation] and make my health and my body strong." Confess that throughout the day whenever you think about your health condition.

Three-Day Juice Fasting Program, Phase I

Consume the juice blend noted here from the time you wake up until 2:00 p.m. Juice is best made fresh in your home juicer. For best results, use organic produce, and consume the juice within twenty minutes of juicing. It is best to consume four eight- to twelve-ounce glasses of the carrot/apple juice blend from the time you wake up until 2:00 p.m.

Juices #1–4: Mix the following in a glass, jar, or hand mixer: four to six ounces carrot juice; four to six ounces apple juice; one tablespoon of powdered digestive enzyme blend (for recommended products, visit www.BiblicalHealthInstitute.com and click on the GPRx Resource Guide)

Three-Day Juice Fasting Program, Phase II

Consume the juice blend noted here from 2:00 p.m. until bedtime. Juice is best made fresh in your home juicer. For best results, use organic produce, and consume the juice within twenty minutes of juicing. It is best to consume four eight- to-twelve-ounce glasses of the carrot/celery/parsley juice blend from 2:00 p.m. until bedtime.

Juices #5–8: Mix the following in a glass, jar, or hand mixer: four-to-six ounces carrot juice; three-to-five ounces celery juice; one-to-two ounces parsley juice; one tablespoon of green super food powder (mixed in) or (swallow) five caplets of green food detoxifying blend (for recommended products, visit www.BiblicalHealthInstitute.com and click on the GPRx Resource Guide).

Before Bed

Body therapy: take a warm bath for fifteen minutes with eight drops of biblical essential oils added. (visit www.BiblicalHealthInstitute.com and click on the GPRx Resource Guide).

Advanced hygiene: repeat the morning advanced hygiene instructions.

Emotional health: ask the Lord to bring to your mind someone you need to forgive. Take out a sheet of paper and write the person's name at the top. Try to remember each specific action that person did against you that brought you pain. Write down the following: "I forgive [insert person's name] for [insert the action he or she did against you]." After you fill up the paper, tear it up or burn it, and ask God to give you the strength to truly forgive that person.

Purpose: ask yourself these questions: *Did I live a life of purpose today? What did I do to add value to someone else's life today?* Commit to living a day of purpose tomorrow.

Prayer: thank God for this day, asking Him to give you a restoring night's rest and a fresh start tomorrow. Thank Him for His steadfast love that never ceases and His mercies new every morning. Read Romans 8:35, 37–39 out loud.

Sleep: go to bed by 10:30 p.m.

DAY 2

Upon Waking and During the Daylight Hours

Prayer: thank God because this is the day that the Lord has made. Rejoice and be glad in it. Thank Him for the breath in your lungs and the life in your body. Ask the Lord to heal your body and use your experience to benefit the lives of others. Read Psalm 91 out loud.

Purpose: ask the Lord to give you an opportunity to add significance to someone's life today. Watch for that opportunity. Ask God to use you this day for His intended purpose.

Advanced hygiene: follow the advanced hygiene recommendations from the morning of Day 1.

Reduce toxins: follow the recommendations to reduce toxins from the morning of Day 1.

Body therapy: take a hot and cold shower. After a normal shower, alternate sixty seconds of water as hot as you can stand it, followed by sixty seconds of water as cold as you can stand it. Repeat cycle four times for a total of eight minutes, finishing with cold.

Exercise: try to walk outside in the fresh air, weather permitting, and finish with five to ten minutes of deep-breathing exercises (if you feel well enough to exercise).

Emotional health: follow the emotional health recommendations from the morning of Day 1.

Three-Day Juice Fasting Program, Phase I

Consume the juice blend noted here from the time you wake up until 2:00 p.m. Juice is best made fresh in your home juicer. For best results, use organic produce, and consume the juice within twenty minutes of juicing. It is best to consume four eight- to twelve-ounce glasses of the carrot/apple juice blend from the time you wake up until 2:00 p.m.

Juices #1–4: Mix the following in a glass, jar, or hand mixer: four to six ounces carrot juice; four to six ounces apple juice; one tablespoon of powdered digestive enzyme blend (for recommended products, visit www.BiblicalHealthInstitute.com and click on the GPRx Resource Guide)

Three-Day Juice Fasting Program, Phase II

Consume the juice blend noted here from 2:00 p.m. until bedtime. Juice is best made fresh in your home juicer. For best results, use organic produce, and consume the juice within twenty minutes of juicing. It is best to consume four eight- to twelve-ounce glasses of the carrot/celery/parsley juice blend from 2:00 p.m. until bedtime.

Juices #5–8: Mix the following in a glass, jar, or hand mixer: four-to-six ounces carrot juice; three-to-five ounces celery juice; one-to-two ounces parsley juice; one tablespoon of green super food powder (mixed in) or (swallow) five caplets of green food detoxifying blend (for recommended products, visit www.BiblicalHealthInstitute.com and click on the GPRx Resource Guide).

Before Bed

Advanced hygiene: follow the advanced hygiene recommendations from the morning of Day 1.

Emotional health: repeat the emotional health recommendations from the evening of Day 1.

Purpose: ask yourself these questions: *Did I live a life of purpose today? What did I do to add value to someone else's life today?* Commit to living a day of purpose tomorrow.

Prayer: thank God for this day, asking Him to give you a restoring night's rest and a fresh start tomorrow. Thank Him for His steadfast love that never ceases and His mercies that are new every morning. Read 1 Corinthians 13:4–8 out loud.

Body therapy: spend ten minutes listening to soothing music before you retire.

Sleep: go to bed by 10:30 p.m.

DAY 3

Upon Waking and During the Daylight Hours

Prayer: thank God because this is the day that the Lord has made. Rejoice and be glad in it. Thank Him for the breath in your lungs and the life in your body. Ask the Lord to heal your body and use your experience to benefit the lives of others. Read Ephesians 6:13–18 out loud.

Purpose: ask the Lord to give you an opportunity to add significance to someone's life today. Watch for that opportunity. Ask God to use you this day for His intended purpose.

Advanced hygiene: follow the advanced hygiene recommendations from the morning of Day 1.

Reduce toxins: follow the recommendations to reduce toxins from the morning of Day 1.

Body therapy: get twenty minutes of direct sunlight sometime during the day, but be careful between the hours of 10:00 a.m. and 2:00 p.m.

Exercise: try to walk outside in the fresh air, weather permitting, and finish with five to ten minutes of deep-breathing exercises (if you feel well enough to exercise).

Emotional health: follow the emotional health recommendations from the morning of Day 1.

Three-Day Juice Fasting Program, Phase I

Consume the juice blend noted here from the time you wake up until 2:00 p.m. Juice is best made fresh in your home juicer. For best results, use organic produce, and consume the juice within twenty minutes of juicing. It is best to consume four eight- to twelve-ounce glasses of the carrot/apple juice blend from the time you wake up until 2:00 p.m.

Juices #1–4: Mix the following in a glass, jar, or hand mixer: four to six ounces carrot juice; four to six ounces apple juice; one tablespoon of powdered digestive enzyme blend (for recommended products, visit www.BiblicalHealthInstitute.com and click on the GPRx Resource Guide)

Three-Day Juice Fasting Program, Phase II

Consume the juice blend noted here from 2:00 p.m. until bedtime. Juice is best made fresh in your home juicer. For best results, use organic produce, and consume the juice within twenty minutes of juicing. It is best to consume four eight- to twelve-ounce glasses of the carrot/celery/parsley juice blend from 2:00 p.m. until bedtime.

Juices #5–8: Mix the following in a glass, jar, or hand mixer: four-to-six ounces carrot juice; three-to-five ounces celery juice; one-to-two ounces parsley juice; one tablespoon of green super food powder (mixed in) or (swallow) five caplets of green food detoxifying blend (for recommended products, visit www.BiblicalHealthInstitute.com and click on the GPRx Resource Guide).

Before Bed

Body therapy: take a warm bath for fifteen minutes with eight drops of biblical essential oils added.

Advanced hygiene: follow the advanced hygiene instructions from the morning of Day 1.

Emotional health: follow the forgiveness recommendations from the evening of Day 1.

Purpose: ask yourself these questions: *Did I live a life of purpose today? What did I do to add value to someone else's life today?* Commit to living a day of purpose tomorrow.

Prayer: thank God for this day, asking Him to give you a restoring night's rest and a fresh start tomorrow. Thank Him for His steadfast love that never ceases and His mercies that are new every morning. Read Philippians 4:4–8, 11–13, 19 out loud.

Sleep: go to bed by 10:30 p.m.

DAY 4

Upon Waking and During the Daylight Hours

Prayer: thank God because this is the day that the Lord has made. Rejoice and be glad in it. Thank Him for the breath in your lungs and the life in your body. Read Matthew 6:9–13 out loud.

Purpose: ask the Lord to give you an opportunity to add significance to someone's life today. Watch for that opportunity. Ask God to use you this day for His intended purpose.

Advanced hygiene: follow the advanced hygiene recommendations from the morning of Day 1.

Reduce toxins: follow the recommendations for reducing toxins from the morning of Day 1.

Morning alkalizing drink: mix two tablespoons of apple cider vinegar and one tablespoon of raw honey into eight to twelve ounces of warm water. Drink slowly and wait for twenty minutes before taking your morning supplements.

Supplements: take one serving of a fiber/green superfood powder (mixed) or five caplets of a super green formula swallowed with twelve-to-sixteen ounces of high-alkaline water or raw vegetable juice. (For recommended products, visit www.BiblicalHealthInstitute.com and click on the GPRx Resource Guide.)

Exercise: perform functional fitness exercises for five to fifteen minutes or spend five to fifteen minutes on a mini trampoline. Finish with five to ten minutes of deep-breathing exercises. (One to three rounds of the exercises can be found at www.Great PhysiciansRx.com.)

Body therapy: take a hot and cold shower. After a normal shower, alternate sixty seconds of water as hot as you can stand it, followed by sixty seconds of water as cold as you can stand it. Repeat cycle four times for a total of eight minutes, finishing with cold.

Emotional health: follow the emotional health recommendations from the morning of Day 1.

Breakfast

Make a smoothie in a blender with the following ingredients: one cup plain yogurt or kefir (goat's milk is best); one tablespoon organic flaxseed oil; one tablespoon organic raw honey; one-half cup organic berries; dash of vanilla extract (optional)

one cup of hot green tea with honey

Supplements: take two whole food multivitamin caplets and two capsules of a probiotic/enzyme blend. (Visit www.BiblicalHealth Institute.com and click on the GPRx Resource Guide for recommendations.)

Lunch

Before eating, drink eight ounces of water.

During lunch, drink eight ounces of water or hot green tea with honey.

large green salad with mixed greens, avocado, carrots, tomatoes, red cabbage, red peppers, and sprouts with two ounces of low mercury, high omega-3 canned tuna

salad dressing: extra virgin olive oil, apple cider vinegar or lemon juice, Celtic sea salt, herbs, and spices one bunch of grapes with seeds

Supplements: take two whole food multivitamin caplets and two capsules of a probiotic/enzyme blend.

Dinner

Before eating, drink eight ounces of water.

During dinner, drink hot green tea with honey.

baked or poached wild-caught salmon

steamed broccoli

large green salad with mixed greens, avocado, carrots, tomatoes, red cabbage, red onions, red peppers, and sprouts

salad dressing: extra virgin olive oil, apple cider vinegar or lemon juice, Celtic sea salt, herbs, and spices

Supplements: take two whole food multivitamin caplets and two capsules of a probiotic/enzyme blend and one-to-three teaspoons or three-to-nine capsules of a high omega-3 cod-liver oil complex. (For recommended products, visit www.BiblicalHealthInstitute.com and click on the GPRx Resource Guide.)

Snacks

apple and carrots with raw almond butter

eight-to-twelve ounces of water, or hot or iced fresh-brewed tea with honey

Before Bed

Drink eight to twelve ounces of water or hot green tea with honey.

Exercise: go for a walk outdoors or participate in a favorite sport or recreational activity.

Supplements: take one serving of a fiber/green superfood powder (mixed) or five caplets of a super green formula swallowed with twelve-to-sixteen ounces of high-alkaline water or raw vegetable juice.

Advanced hygiene: follow the advanced hygiene recommendations from the morning of Day 1.

Emotional health: follow the forgiveness recommendations from the evening of Day 1.

Purpose: ask yourself these questions: *Did I live a life of purpose today? What did I do to add value to someone else's life today?* Commit to living a day of purpose tomorrow.

Prayer: thank God for this day, asking Him to give you a restoring night's rest and a fresh start tomorrow. Thank Him for His steadfast love that never ceases and His mercies that are new every morning. Read Romans 8:35, 37–39 out loud.

Body therapy: spend ten minutes listening to soothing music before you retire.

Sleep: go to bed by 10:30 p.m.

DAY 5 (PARTIAL-FAST DAY)

Upon Waking

Prayer: thank God because this is the day that the Lord has made. Rejoice and be glad in it. Thank Him for the breath in your lungs and the life in your body. Read Isaiah 58:6–9 out loud.

Purpose: ask the Lord to give you an opportunity to add significance to someone's life today. Watch for that opportunity. Ask God to use you this day for His intended purpose.

Advanced hygiene: follow the advanced hygiene recommendations from the morning of Day 1.

Reduce toxins: follow the recommendations for reducing toxins from the morning of Day 1.

Morning alkalizing drink: mix two tablespoons of apple cider vinegar and one tablespoon of raw honey into eight-to-twelve ounces of warm water. Drink slowly and wait for twenty minutes before taking your morning supplements.

Supplements: take one serving of a fiber/green superfood powder (mixed) or five caplets of a super green formula swallowed with twelve-to-sixteen ounces of high-alkaline water or raw vegetable juice.

Exercise: perform functional fitness exercises for five to fifteen minutes or spend five to fifteen minutes on a mini trampoline. Finish with five to ten minutes of deep-breathing exercises. (One to three rounds of the exercises can be found at www.GreatPhysiciansRx.com.)

Body therapy: get twenty minutes of direct sunlight sometime during the day, but be careful between the hours of 10:00 a.m. and 2:00 p.m.

Emotional health: follow the emotional health recommendations from the morning of Day 1.

Breakfast

none (partial-fast day)

eight to twelve ounces of vegetable juice or high-alkaline water

Supplements: take two capsules of a probiotic/enzyme blend.

Lunch

none (partial-fast day)

eight ounces of vegetable juice or high-alkaline water

Supplements: take two capsules of a probiotic/enzyme blend.

Dinner

Before eating, drink eight ounces of water.

During dinner, drink hot green tea with honey.

Chicken Soup (visit www.GreatPhysiciansRx.com for the recipe)

cultured vegetables

large green salad with mixed greens, avocado, carrots, tomatoes, red cabbage, red onions, red peppers, and sprouts salad dressing: extra virgin olive oil, apple cider vinegar or lemon juice, Celtic sea salt, herbs, and spices

Supplements: take six whole food multivitamin caplets and two capsules of a probiotic/enzyme blend and one-to-three teaspoons or three-to-nine capsules of a high omega-3 cod-liver oil complex.

Snacks
none (partial-fast day)

eight ounces of water

Before Bed
Drink eight to twelve ounces of water or hot green tea with honey.

Exercise: go for a walk outdoors or participate in a favorite sport or recreational activity.

Supplements: take one serving of a fiber/green superfood powder (mixed) or five caplets of a super green formula swallowed with twelve-to-sixteen ounces of high-alkaline water or raw vegetable juice.

Advanced hygiene: follow the advanced hygiene recommendations from the morning of Day 1.

Emotional health: follow the forgiveness recommendations from the evening of Day 1.

Body therapy: take a warm bath for fifteen minutes with eight drops of biblical essential oils added.

Purpose: ask yourself these questions: *Did I live a life of purpose today? What did I do to add value to someone else's life today?* Commit to living a day of purpose tomorrow.

Prayer: thank God for this day, asking Him to give you a restoring night's rest and a fresh start tomorrow. Thank Him for His steadfast love that never ceases and His mercies that are new every morning. Read Isaiah 58:6–9 out loud.

Sleep: go to bed by 10:30 p.m.

DAY 6 (REST DAY)

Upon Waking

Prayer: thank God because this is the day that the Lord has made. Rejoice and be glad in it. Thank Him for the breath in your lungs and the life in your body. Read Psalm 23 out loud.

Purpose: ask the Lord to give you an opportunity to add significance to someone's life today. Watch for that opportunity. Ask God to use you this day for His intended purpose.

Advanced hygiene: follow the advanced hygiene recommendations from the morning of Day 1.

Reduce toxins: follow the recommendations for reducing toxins from the morning of Day 1.

Morning alkalizing drink: mix two tablespoons of apple cider vinegar and one tablespoon of raw honey into eight-to-twelve ounces of warm water. Drink slowly and wait for twenty minutes before taking your morning supplements.

Supplements: take one serving of a fiber/green superfood powder (mixed) or five caplets of a super green formula swallowed with twelve-to-sixteen ounces of high-alkaline water or raw vegetable juice.

Exercise: no formal exercise since it's a rest day.

Body therapies: none since it's a rest day.

Emotional health: follow emotional health recommendations from the morning of Day 1.

Breakfast

one cup of hot green tea with honey

Make a smoothie in a blender with the following ingredients:

one cup plain yogurt or kefir (goat's milk is best)

one tablespoon organic flaxseed oil

one tablespoon organic raw honey

one-half cup organic berries

dash of vanilla extract (optional)

Supplements: take two whole food multivitamin caplets and two capsules of a probiotic/enzyme blend.

Lunch

Before eating, drink eight ounces of water.

During lunch, drink eight ounces of water or hot green tea with honey.

large green salad with mixed greens, avocado, carrots, tomatoes, red cabbage, red onions, red peppers, and sprouts with three ounces of cold poached or canned wild salmon

salad dressing: extra virgin olive oil, apple cider vinegar or lemon juice, Celtic sea salt, herbs, and spices

one organic apple with the skin

Supplements: take two whole food multivitamin caplets and two capsules of a probiotic/enzyme blend.

Dinner

Before eating, drink eight ounces of water.

During dinner, drink hot green tea with honey.

roasted organic chicken

cooked vegetables (carrots, onions, peas, etc.)

large green salad with mixed greens, avocado, carrots, tomatoes, red cabbage, red onions, red peppers, and sprouts

salad dressing: extra virgin olive oil, apple cider vinegar or lemon juice, Celtic sea salt, herbs, and spices

Supplements: take six whole food multivitamin caplets and two capsules of a probiotic/enzyme blend and one-to-three teaspoons or three-to-nine capsules of a high omega-3 cod-liver oil complex.

Snacks

   raw almonds

   one apple

   eight-to-twelve ounces of water, or hot or iced fresh-brewed tea with honey

Before Bed

   Drink eight-to-twelve ounces of water or hot tea with honey.

   Exercise: go for a walk outdoors or participate in a favorite sport or recreational activity.

   Supplements: take one serving of a fiber/green superfood powder (mixed) or five caplets of a super green formula swallowed with twelve-to-sixteen ounces of high-alkaline water or raw vegetable juice.

   Advanced hygiene: follow the advanced hygiene recommendations from the morning of Day 1.

   Emotional health: follow the forgiveness recommendations from the evening of Day 1.

   Purpose: ask yourself these questions: *Did I live a life of purpose today? What did I do to add value to someone else's life today?* Commit to living a day of purpose tomorrow.

   Prayer: thank God for this day, asking Him to give you a restoring night's rest and a fresh start tomorrow. Thank Him for His steadfast love that never ceases and His mercies that are new every morning. Read Psalm 23 out loud.

   Body therapy: spend ten minutes listening to soothing music before you retire.

   Sleep: go to bed by 10:30 p.m.

Day 7

Upon Waking

   Prayer: thank God because this is the day that the Lord has made.

Rejoice and be glad in it. Thank Him for the breath in your lungs and the life in your body. Read Psalm 91 out loud.

Purpose: ask the Lord to give you an opportunity to add significance to someone's life today. Watch for that opportunity. Ask God to use you this day for His intended purpose.

Advanced hygiene: follow the advanced hygiene recommendations from the morning of Day 1.

Reduce toxins: follow the recommendations for reducing toxins from the morning of Day 1.

Morning alkalizing drink: mix two tablespoons of apple cider vinegar and one tablespoon of raw honey into eight-to-twelve ounces of warm water. Drink slowly and wait for twenty minutes before taking your morning supplements.

Supplements: take one serving of a fiber/green superfood powder (mixed) or five caplets of a super green formula swallowed with twelve-to-sixteen ounces of high-alkaline water or raw vegetable juice.

Exercise: perform functional fitness exercises for five to fifteen minutes or spend five to fifteen minutes on a mini trampoline. Finish with five to ten minutes of deep-breathing exercises. (One to three rounds of the exercises can be found at www.GreatPhysiciansRx.com.)

Body therapy: get twenty minutes of direct sunlight sometime during the day, but be careful between the hours of 10:00 a.m. and 2:00 p.m.

Emotional health: follow the emotional health recommendations from the morning of Day 1.

Breakfast

Make a smoothie in a blender with the following ingredients: one cup plain yogurt or kefir (goat's milk is best); one tablespoon organic flaxseed oil; one tablespoon organic raw honey; one cup organic fruit (berries, banana, peaches, pineapple, etc.); two tablespoons goat's milk protein powder; dash of vanilla extract (optional)

Supplements: take two whole food multivitamin caplets and two capsules of a probiotic/enzyme blend.

Lunch

Before eating, drink eight ounces of water.

During lunch, drink eight ounces of water or hot green tea with honey.

large green salad with mixed greens, avocado, tomatoes, carrots, red cabbage, red peppers, and sprouts with one hard-boiled omega-3 egg

salad dressing: extra virgin olive oil, apple cider vinegar or lemon juice, Celtic sea salt, herbs, and spices

one piece of fruit in season

Supplements: take two whole food multivitamin caplets and two capsules of a probiotic/enzyme blend.

Dinner

Before eating, drink eight ounces of water.

During dinner, drink hot green tea with honey.

baked or poached wild-caught salmon

steamed broccoli

large green salad with mixed greens, avocado, carrots, tomatoes, red cabbage, red onions, red peppers, and sprouts

salad dressing: extra virgin olive oil, apple cider vinegar or lemon juice, Celtic sea salt, herbs, and spices

Supplements: take six whole food multivitamin caplets and two capsules of a probiotic/enzyme blend and one to three teaspoons or three to nine capsules of a high omega-3 cod liver oil complex.

Snacks

apple slices with raw sesame butter (tahini)

eight-to-twelve ounces of water, or hot or iced fresh-brewed tea with honey

Before Bed

Drink eight-to-twelve ounces of water or hot tea with honey.

Exercise: go for a walk outdoors or participate in a favorite sport or recreational activity.

Supplements: take one serving of a fiber/green superfood powder (mixed) or five caplets of a super green formula swallowed with twelve-to-sixteen ounces of high-alkaline water or raw vegetable juice.

Advanced hygiene: follow the advanced hygiene recommendations from the morning of Day 1.

Emotional health: follow the forgiveness recommendations from the evening of Day 1.

Body therapy: take a warm bath for fifteen minutes with eight drops of biblical essential oils added.

Purpose: ask yourself these questions: "Did I live a life of purpose today?" "What did I do to add value to someone else's life today?" Commit to living a day of purpose tomorrow.

Prayer: thank God for this day, asking Him to give you a restoring night's rest and a fresh start tomorrow. Thank Him for His steadfast love that never ceases and His mercies that are new every morning. Read 1 Corinthians 13:4–8 out loud.

Sleep: go to bed by 10:30 p.m.

Day 8 and Beyond

If you're beginning to feel better, but still have a way to go on your road to wellness, you can repeat the Great Physician's Rx for Cancer Battle Plan as many times as you'd like. If you are feeling better but want to continue on an extremely healthy lifestyle, follow the basic guidelines for Day 7 while changing your exercise, prayer, and meal plans each day.

For detailed step-by-step suggestions, meals, and lifestyle plans, visit www.GreatPhysiciansRx.com and join the Lifetime of Wellness plan. This online program will provide you with customized daily meals and exercise planning and provide you with tools to track your progress.

If you've experienced positive results from the Great Physician's Rx for Cancer program, I encourage you to reach out to others you know and recommend this book and program to them. You don't have to be a doctor or a health expert to help transform the lives of people you care about.

Allow me to offer this prayer of blessing from Numbers 6:24–26 for you:

May the Lord bless you and keep you.
May the Lord make His face to shine upon you and be
    gracious unto you.
May the Lord lift up His countenance upon you and bring
    you peace.
In the name of Yeshua Ha Mashiach, Jesus our Messiah.
Amen.

Need Recipes?

For a detailed list of more than two hundred healthy and delicious recipes contained in the Great Physician's Rx eating plan, please visit www.GreatPhysiciansRx.com.

NOTES

Introduction

1. American Cancer Society, *Cancer Facts & Figures 2005* (Atlanta: American Cancer Society, 2005).

2. "Who Gets Cancer?" American Cancer Society Web site, http://www.cancer.org/docroot/CRI/content/CRI_2_4_1x_Who_gets _cancer.asp?sitearea=.

3. "Annual Report to the Nation on the Status of Cancer, 1975 to 2001," released in June 2004. The annual cancer report is a collaborative effort by the National Cancer Institute, the American Cancer Society, the federal Centers for Disease Control and Prevention, and the North American Association of Central Cancer Registries.

4. "The History of Cancer," medicineworld.org, http://www.medicineworld.org/cancer/history.html.

5. *The Encyclopedia of Nutritional Healing* (Burnaby, BC, Canada: Alive Publishing Group, Inc., 1997), 247.

6. Ibid..

7. http://www.hopkinshospital.org/health_info/Cancer/Reading/ alternative_cancer_treatments.html.

8. From http://www.quackwatch.org/01QuackeryRelatedTopics/ Cancer/laetrile.html.

Key #1

1. Committee on Diet, Nutrition, and Cancer, Assembly of Life Sciences, National Research Council, *Diet, Nutrition, and Cancer* (Washington, D.C.: National Academy Press, 1982).

2. Dr. Johanna Budwig, *Flax Oil as a True Aid Against Arthritis, Heart Infarction, Cancer, and Other Diseases* (Canada: Apple Publishing, 1994).

3. Dr. Appleton listed three sources for this dramatic statement: A. Sanchez et al., "Role of Sugars in Human Neutrophilic Phagocytosis," *American Journal of Clinical Nutrition* 261 (November 1973): 1180–84; J. Bernstein et al., "Depression of Lymphocyte Transformation Following Oral Glucose Ingestion," *American Journal of Clinical Nutrition* 30 (1997): 613; and W. Ringsdorf, E. Cheraskin, and R. Ramsay, "Sucrose, Neutrophilic Phagocytosis and Resistance to Disease," *Dental Survey* 52 (1976): 46–48.

4. Environmental News Service, "Honey Bee Products Potent in Cancer Prevention, Treatment," December 7, 2004, http://www.keepmedia.com/pubs/EnvironmentNewsService/2004/12/07/677614?from=search&criteria=Honey+Bee+products+in+Cancer&refinePubTypeID=0.

5. Maureen Keane, M.S., and Daniella Chace, M.S., "Carbohydrates and Cancer," WebMD Medical Reference, "What to Eat if You Have Cancer," http://my.webmd.com/content/article/83/97645.htm.

6. T. Norat, *Journal of the National Cancer Institute,* June 15, 2005, 906–16, news release, National Cancer Institute, http://my.webmd.com/content/article/107/108494.htm.

7. *The Health Effects of Nitrate, Nitrite, and N-Nitroso Compounds* (Washington, D.C.: National Academy of Sciences, 1981).

8. P. Tonilo et al., "Consumption of Meat, Animal Products, Protein and Fat and Risk of Breast Cancer: A Prospective Cohort Study in New York," *Epidemiology* 5, no. 4 (1994): 391.

9. Karla Gale, "Pomegranate Juice Promising for Prostate Cancer," Reuters News Service, September 26, 2005, http://today.reuters.com/news/newsArticle.aspx?type=healthNews&storyID=2005-09-26T223623Z_01_HAR681364_RTRUKOC_0_US-POMEGRANATE-CANCER.xml&archived=False.

10. "Green Tea Can Block Cancer," BBC World News, August 5, 2003, http://news.bbc.co.uk/1/hi/health/3125469.stm.

11. Kathleen Doheny, "Curry Spice Shuts Down Melanoma," *HealthDay*, July 11, 2005, based on research by University of Texas M. D. Anderson Cancer Center, Houston, Texas.

12. Y. K. Surh, E. Lee, and J. M. Lee, "Chemoprotective Properties of Some Pungent Ingredients of Red Pepper and Ginger," *Mutat Res* 402, nos. 1–2 (June 18, 1998): 259–67.

13. F. Batmanghelidj, M.D., *You're Not Sick, You're Thirsty!* (New York: Warner Books, 2003), 218. For articles related to drinking water and cancer, see www.watercure.com.

14. "Alcohol Alert," National Institute on Alcohol Abuse and Alcoholism, no. 21 PH 345, July 1993, http://www.niaaa.nih.gov/publications/aa21.htm.

Key #2

1. W. Elaine Hardman, "Omega-3 Fatty Acids to Augment Cancer Therapy," *Journal of Nutrition* 132 (November 2002): 3508S–3512S.

2. "Tea Looks Promising as Cancer Fighter," University of Virginia Health System, http://www.healthsystem.virginia.edu/uvahealth/news_mindbody/0406mb.cfm.

3. "Green Tea Can Block Cancer," BBC World News Bulletin, August 5, 2003, http://news.bbc.co.uk/2/hi/health/3125469.stm.

4. Warren Froelich, "Fruits Offer Powerful Protection from Skin Cancer," American Association for Cancer Research, October 29, 2003, http://www.aacr.org/Default.aspx?p=2084&d=190.

5. "Antimicrobial and Chemopreventive Properties of Herbs and Spices," *Current Medical Chemistry*, June 2004, 1451–60, http://www.ncbi.nlm.nih.gov/entrez/query.fcgi?cmd=Retrieve&db=pubmed&dopt=Abstract&list_uids=15180577.

6. "Common Essential Mineral May Reduce the Risk of Some Cancers," *Los Angeles Times*, July 4, 2005.

7. "Pharmacy Island," *Newsweek*'s special edition of "Your Health in the 21st Century," Summer 2005, 58.

8. The entire list, with the exception of beta-carotene, comes from *The Side Effects Bible* by Frederic Vagnani, M.D., and Barry Fox, Ph.D. (New York: Broadway Books, 2005).

Key #3

1. Carol M. Ostrom, "The Circumcision Decision: Merits of Procedure Debated," *Seattle Times*, July 9, 2003.

2. Neil Osterweil, "Circumcising Newborns May Protect Against Penile Cancer," WebMD Medical News, http://my.webmd.com/content/article/22/1728_55462.htm.

3. "Male Circumcision, Penile Human Papillomavirus Infection, and Cervical Cancer in Female Partners," *New England Journal of Medicine*, April 2002, Volume 346:1105–1112, Number 15, http://content.nejm.org/cgi/content/abstract/346/15/1105.>

4. "New Study Shows Benefit of Male Circumcision," June 4, 2002, WebMD Web site, http://www.cancer.org/docroot/NWS/content/NWS_1_1x_New_Study_Shows_Benefit_of_Male_Circumcision.asp.

5. "New Breast Cancer Drug Approved," *American Cancer Society News*, January 12, 2005, http://health.yahoo.com/news/54426.

Key #4

1. Holmes et al., "Physical Activity and Survival After Breast Cancer Diagnosis," JAMA, 2005; 293: 2479-2486.

2. "Exercise Reduces Risk of Recurrence and Death in Early Stage Colon Cancer Patients," a press release issued May 17, 2005 by the Dana-Farber Cancer Institute and available at http://www.dana-farber.org/abo/news/press/exercise-reduces-risk-colon-cancer.asp.

3. Amanda Gardner, "Lifestyle Can Dictate Course of Breast Cancer," *HealthDay*, June 9, 2005.

4. "Physical Exercise," Stanford Cancer Center Web site, http://cancer.stanfordhospital.com/healthInfo/alternativeTherapy/exercise/default.

5. D. Greene, L. M. Nail, V. K. Fieler, et al., "A Comparison of Patient-Reported Side Effects Among Three Chemotherapy Regimens for Cancer," *Cancer Pract* 2, no. 1 (1994): 57–62.

6. "Link Between Sleep, Cancer Progression Explored by Stanford Researcher," a news release issued February 13, 2004 by the Stanford School of Medicine, and available at http://mednews.stanford.edu/releases/2004/february/AAASSpiegel.htm.

7. Joan Raymond and Jerry Adler, "A Neglected Nutrient: Are Americans Dying from a Lack of Vitamin D?" *Newsweek,* January 17, 2005.

8. Alex Raksin, "Making a Case for Sun's Benefit's," *Los Angeles Times,* June 20, 2005.

9. Marilynn Marchione, "Scientists Say Sunshine May Prevent Cancer," MyWay Web site, May 21, 2005, http://apnews.myway.com/article/20050521/D8A7PB5O0.html>.

10. *The Encyclopedia of Natural Healing* (Burnaby, BC: Alive Publishing Group, 1997), 559.

Key #5
1. "Body Burden: The Pollution in People," Environmental Working Group report, January 2003. (A complete rundown of this landmark 2003 study can be found at www.ewg.org/reports/bodyburden/es.php.)

2. Ibid.

3. David Steinman and Samuel S. Epstein, M.D., *The Safe Shopper's Bible* (New York: Wiley Publishing, 1995), 18.

Key #6
1. Steven Locke et al., "Life Change Stress, Psychiatric Symptoms, and Natural Killer Activity," *Psychosomatic Medicine* 46, no. 5 (1984): 441–53.

Key #7
1. Germaine Copeland, *Prayers That Avail Much* (Tulsa, OK: Harrison House, 1997), 104–5.

About the Authors

Jordan Rubin has dedicated his life to transforming the health of others one life at a time. He is the founder and chairman of Garden of Life, Inc., a health and wellness company based in West Palm Beach, Florida, that produces whole food nutritional supplements and personal care products. He is also president and CEO of GPRx, Inc., a biblically based health and wellness company providing educational resources, small group curriculum, functional foods, nutritional supplements, and wellness services.

He and his wife, Nicki, married in 1999 and are the parents of a toddler-aged son, Joshua. They make their home in Palm Beach Gardens, Florida.

Joseph D. Brasco, M.D., who is board certified in internal medicine and gastroenterology, is in private practice in Indianapolis, Indiana. He has skillfully combined diet, supplementation, and judicious use of medications to provide a comprehensive and effective treatment program. Dr. Brasco is the coauthor of *Restoring Your Digestive Health* with Jordan Rubin.

The Great Physician's Rx DVD and Study Guide

LEARN AND APPLY 7 TIPS TO GOOD HEALTH

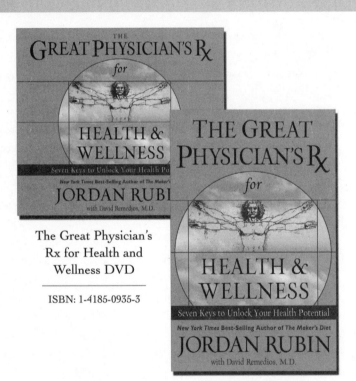

The Great Physician's
Rx for Health and
Wellness DVD

ISBN: 1-4185-0935-3

NELSON IMPACT
A Division of Thomas Nelson Publishers
Since 1798

www.thomasnelson.com

The Great Physician's
Rx for Health and
Wellness Study Guide

ISBN: 1-4185-0934-5

BHI

BIBLICAL HEALTH
INSTITUTE

The Biblical Health Institute (www.BiblicalHealthInstitute.com) is an online learning community housing educational resources and curricula reinforcing and expanding on Jordan Rubin's Biblical Health message.

Biblical Health Institute provides:

1. "101" level **FREE**, introductory courses corresponding to Jordan's book The Great Physician's Rx for Health and Wellness and its seven keys; Current "101" courses include:

   * "Eating to Live 101"

   * "Whole Food Nutrition Supplements 101"

   * "Advanced Hygiene 101"

   * "Exercise and Body Therapies 101"

   * "Reducing Toxins 101"

   * "Emotional Health 101"

   * "Prayer and Purpose 101"

2. **FREE** resources (healthy recipes, what to E.A.T., resource guide)

3. **FREE** media--videos and video clips of Jordan, music therapy samples, etc.--and much more!

Additionally, Biblical Health Institute also offers in-depth courses for those who want to go deeper.

Course offerings include:

   * 40-hour certificate program to become a Biblical Health Coach

   * A la carte course offerings designed for personal study and growth (launching late April 2006)

   * Home school courses developed by Christian educators, supporting home-schooled students and their parents (designed for middle school and high school ages—launching in August 2006).

**For more information and updates on these and other resources go to
www.BiblicalHealthInstitute.com**

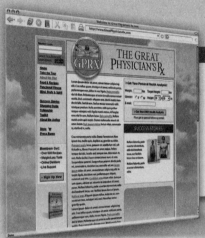

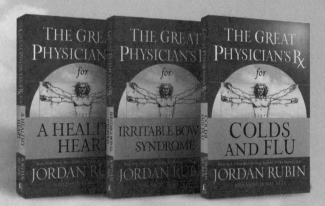

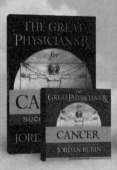
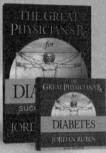
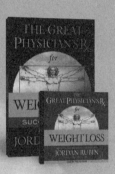